THE DOCTORS BOOK
OF
Home Remedies®
FOR
MANAGING MENOPAUSE

More Than 100 Solutions for Conquering Symptoms and Facing the Future with Confidence

By the Editors of *PREVENTION.*
Edited by Mary S. Kittel

RODALE

Printed in the United States of America
Rodale Inc. makes every effort to use acid-free ∞,
recycled paper ♻ .

Illustrations: Karen Kuchar and Judy Newhouse (p. 63)
Cover Design: Lynn N. Gano and Tara Long
Cover Photograph: Rodale Images

Library of Congress Cataloging-in-Publication Data

The doctors book of home remedies for managing menopause : more than 100 solutions for conquering symptoms and facing the future with confidence / by the editors of Prevention ; edited by Mary S. Kittel.
      p.   cm.
   Includes index.
   ISBN 1–57954–234–4 paperback
   1. Menopause—Alternative treatment.   2. Middle aged women—Health and hygiene.   3. Self-care, Health.   I. Kittel, Mary S.   II. Prevention (Emmaus, Pa.)
RG186 .D635   2001
618.1'7506—dc21   00–009751

Distributed to the book trade by St. Martin's Press

2   4   6   8   10   9   7   5   3   1   paperback

Visit us on the Web at www.rodaleremedies.com,
or call us toll-free at (800) 848-4735.

About *Prevention* Health Books

The editors of *Prevention* Health Books are dedicated to providing you with authoritative, trustworthy, and innovative advice for a healthy, active lifestyle. In all of our books, our goal is to keep you thoroughly informed about the latest breakthroughs in natural healing, medical research, alternative health, herbs, nutrition, fitness, and weight loss. We cut through the confusion of today's conflicting health reports to deliver clear, concise, and definitive health information that you can trust. And we explain in practical terms what each new breakthrough means to you, so you can take immediate, practical steps to improve your health and well-being.

Every recommendation in *Prevention* Health Books is based upon interviews with highly qualified health authorities, including medical doctors and practitioners of alternative medicine. In addition, we consult with the *Prevention* Health Books Board of Advisors to ensure that all of the health information is safe, practical, and up-to-date. *Prevention* Health Books are thoroughly factchecked for accuracy, and we make every effort to verify recommendations, dosages, and cautions.

The advice in this book will help keep you well-informed about your personal choices in health care—to help you lead a happier, healthier, and longer life.

Notice

This book is intended as a reference volume only, not as a medical manual. The information given here is designed to help you make informed decisions about your health. It is not intended as a substitute for any treatment that may have been prescribed by your doctor. If you suspect that you have a medical problem, we urge you to seek competent medical help.

The prescriptions in this book are meant to be followed specifically as given. Unless you are advised by a qualified practitioner, do not take higher dosages, mix the remedies with medications, or use the recommended herbs, essential oils, or supplements during pregnancy or while nursing. Always check with your doctor before beginning a new exercise program or if you experience any unfavorable reaction to a home remedy.

Titles in
The Doctors Book of Home Remedies
series

Acknowledgments

Writers: Barbara Boughton, Laura Catalano, Bob Condor, Kara Messinger, Colleen Pierre, R.D.
Contributing Editor: Doug Dollemore
Editorial Researchers: Shelby Evans, Holly Ann Swanson

We would like to thank the following professionals for their health and wellness advice: Lawrence J. Appel, M.D.; Claudette Baker, L.Ac.; Toni Bark, M.D.; Barbara D. Bartlik, M.D.; Kenneth I. Burke, R.D., Ph.D.; Felicia Busch, R.D.; Don Campbell; Linda De Villers, Ph.D.; Alice D. Domar, Ph.D.; Michele Wheat Dugan; Victoria Edwards, R.N.; Peggy Elam, Ph.D.; Gerald Epstein, M.D.; Mary P. Faine, R.D.; Trisha Lamb Feuerstein; Gail Frank, R.D., Dr.P.H.; Tracy Gaudet, M.D.; Bob Goldman, M.D.; Barbara Gollman, R.D.; Sadja Greenwood, M.D.; Jesse Hanley, M.D.; Clare M. Hasler, Ph.D.; JoAnn Hattner, R.D.; Louise Hay; Helen Healy, N.D.; Edith Howard Hogan, R.D.; Martha Howard, M.D.; Tori Hudson, N.D.; Susan Jeffers, Ph.D.; Elzbieta M. Kurowska, Ph.D.; Loren G. Lipson, M.D.; Patricia Love, Ed.D.; Beth Miller; Mary Jane Minkin, M.D.; Doron Nassimiha, M.D.; Jackie Newgent, R.D.; Karen Nichols, D.O.; David Nickel, O.M.D., L.Ac.; Nadine Pazder, R.D.; Linda Rado; Sheah Rarback, R.D.; Domeena C. Renshaw, M.D.; Christine Rosenbloom, R.D., Ph.D.; Mona Shangold, M.D.; David Simon, M.D.; Heather H. Thomas, Ph.D.; Cyndi Thomson, R.D., Ph.D.; Yvonne S. Thornton, M.D.; Varro Tyler, Ph.D.; Brian Walsh, M.D.; Liz Ward, R.D.; Densie Webb, R.D., Ph.D.; Walter Willett, M.D., Dr.P.H.; Kimberly Windstar, N.D.; David Winston; Laura Yochum, R.D.; Janet Zand, O.M.D., L.Ac.; Kathleen Zelman, R.D.

Contents

Here's what you need to consider when planning a transition out of your reproductive years to facilitate maximum health and minimum stress. Discover that, by creating a personal strategy, what awaits you is quite possibly the most liberating and fulfilling time of life. Experts overview crucial self-care considerations, from the pros and cons of hormone-replacement therapy to the importance of attitude, disease prevention, and exercise.

Did you know that snacking on oranges can lower your cholesterol but that dipping into salsa can summon those evil hot flashes? Try delightful recipes and nutrition tips that can help you not only control symptoms but also lower risks for cancer, cardiovascular disease, osteoporosis, and other diseases associated with aging.

As your hormones adjust, a few physical symptoms are to be expected. For some women, it's hot flashes, and for others, it's fatigue or heavy menstrual bleeding. Our experts will prepare you with powerful solutions that gently nurture and restore your body—from insomnia-curing herbal formulas to night-sweat-stopping breathing techniques. Also, look for cut-to-the-chase tips on fighting flab.

MANAGING YOUR MANY MOODS 69

For the majority of women, menopause is a passage of life worth celebrating. But if you are experiencing grief or anxiety, experts will offer specific pointers on transforming emotional turbulence into peace and self-discovery. Here are steps to becoming the most courageous, creative, and energetic woman you ever wanted to be.

SAVORING SEX 99

Sex therapists and other authorities reveal how to achieve the kind of intimacy that was worth waiting 50 years for. By giving your reproductive system some extra care, you won't have to experience age-related sexual issues like flagging libido, painful intercourse, or increased infections. Experts candidly discuss everything from body image to new adventures in bed.

ALTERNATIVE OPTIONS 121

Alternative medicine draws on techniques from around the world to ease your transition. This directory guides you to the healers who harness ancient and cutting edge cures for women's concerns—including acupuncturists, naturopathic doctors, massage therapists, and more.

INDEX 129

Making a Smooth Change

Expect the Best

Her life began on Parisian streets as an orphan, so destitute and overlooked that she never knew her age. But Gabrielle "Coco" Chanel earned herself a permanent place in the world's most exclusive fashion circles by revolutionizing dress design with the simple glamour of "the Chanel look." Although she chose to leave the fashion scene at middle age, Chanel later made a postretirement comeback so swashbuckling that it inspired a Broadway play.

Anna Mary Robertson was to become a one-room-schoolhouse-educated farmer's wife, whose spare time was absorbed by embroidery. When arthritis forced her to abandon this passion at age 76, she taught herself to paint. By the age of 101, she had produced 600 paintings and was known as darling of the folk art world, Grandma Moses.

Clara McBride Hale became known throughout Harlem, New York, for raising 30 displaced youngsters in addition to her own children. Understanding the special needs of children from drug-addicted mothers, she founded Harlem's Hale House in her seventies, which, under her daughter's direction, continues to provide love and medical attention to hundreds of underprivileged babies.

It's no wonder that cultural anthropologist Margaret Mead declared, "the most creative force in the world is a menopausal woman with zest."

At the age of 72, Mead herself was elected president of the American Association for the Advancement of Science, where she continued researching solutions to worldwide gender and economic inequalities for 5 more years.

But it's not just women in the limelight who discovered their largest potential to create, advocate, teach, and "live zestfully," far beyond their fifties.

Consider the baby-boomer-and-beyond women you know who are shaping the future in wildly rambunctious or quietly dedicated ways. Consider your own seeds of ambition and the blooms you have yet to color the world with. A few hot flashes are hardly enough to disrupt this force.

In survey after survey sponsored by the North American Menopause Society, women consistently report that their menopausal years are the most fulfilling and happiest of their lives. Close to 80 percent of women say that cessation of menstruation came as a relief. More than half say that reaching menopause was a positive turning point in their lives. They reported having more time and energy to focus on hobbies, relationships, and other interests. And three out of four made some type of health-related improvement such as finally quitting smoking. Only 11 percent of the women reported that menopause was a negative experience.

But these outcomes aren't merely luck of the draw. Preventing and alleviating complications from menopause is about taking advantage of today's vast resources and options. That is what this book is all about. Every page will empower you to healthfully and heartily journey into a new and fulfilling stage of life. Despite the fact that history sometimes makes menopause out to be a liability, you will soon learn that it can actually be an opportunity.

Knowledge Is Power

"When perimenopause hit me, it took a few months for my body and mind to adjust," says Kimberly Windstar, N.D., a faculty member at the National College of Naturopathic

Medicine and a naturopathic physician at New Health Horizons clinic, both in Portland, Oregon. "But the better prepared you are, mentally and physically, the smoother the transition is likely to be."

During perimenopause, which occurs in the 3 to 5 years before their final menstrual cycles, most women experience some menstrual irregularities and other symptoms. Menopause is defined as the time when ovaries stop functioning and menstruation ceases. It punctuates the end of a woman's reproductive years, though the process is gradual. Women are categorized as postmenopausal after 12 consecutive months of missed periods.

At menopause, an average American woman is 51 years old. Most women—60 to 80 percent—experience only mild to moderate discomfort during menopause. About 10 to 20 percent have virtually no symptoms at all. For the remaining 10 to 20 percent, the experience is, at best, annoying and, at worst, incapacitating.

The major physiological marker for menopause is a significant decrease of estrogen in a woman's body. A postmenopausal woman's estrogen production is about one-third of what it was during her childbearing years. This drop can cause the side effects widely associated with perimenopause and menopause: hot flashes, night sweats, sleep problems, heavy or irregular menstrual bleeding, weight gain, irritability, forgetfulness, and fatigue.

"The most important thing I tell women about menopausal complications is that they will survive," says Karen Nichols, D.O., an osteopathic physician and director of Southwest Medical Associates in Mesa, Arizona. "So many patients come to me saying that their lives are out of control, that they are wrecks physically and emotionally. They need to hear that everything will be okay—and it will." Remember that the worst is over for most women in only a few months to a year.

Think of any turbulence you may experience at the onset as ultimately a process freeing you from a lifetime of hormone fluctuations. And with medical advancements and traditional folk remedies, hormone researchers and self-help visionaries, you have a wealth of support in adjusting with maximum health and minimum stress.

Getting Personal: The HRT Choice

Many experts in women's health mark the implementation of hormone-replacement therapy (HRT) drugs in the 1940s as the beginning of a liberating revolution in which women can now control their long-term health risks and short-term discomforts of menopause. Others sorely see the medication as unjustified medical intervention that treats a natural process like a disease.

Slightly less than half of American menopausal women use HRT while the second half chooses natural alternatives or none. Taking hormones during menopause and beyond certainly has its advantages. It can eliminate or reduce hot flashes and night sweats, while cutting down on irritability and depression. It also protects against vaginal dryness and aging of the skin. Some women rave about the role of HRT in maintaining their sex lives.

What's more, estrogen is a proven agent for preventing bone loss and regulating cholesterol. So hormone replacement can be especially valuable for any woman with a family history of osteoporosis, heart disease, and stroke. Research findings also show that women taking estrogen have a 54 percent lower risk for Alzheimer's disease compared with women who have never taken the hormone supplement. Some studies indicate that taking estrogen also fights colon cancer.

But the treatment might also increase the risk for breast cancer and cause unwanted side effects that greatly alter the quality of life for some women, such as unpredictable menstrual bleeding, bloating, breast tenderness, headaches, nausea, and mood swings.

A woman's decision regarding hormone-replacement therapy isn't getting any easier either. Two prominent studies in the late 1990s came down on opposite sides of whether the typical hormone-replacement therapy of estrogen and progesterone can lead to increased risk for breast cancer. One study made front-page news by indicating that postmenopausal women on hormonal treatment should have no concerns about breast cancer, while the other showed that taking a combination of estrogen and progesterone increases breast cancer risk by 80 percent.

Count on Your Women's Wisdom

Should you take medication or not? What tests should you put yourself through? Where do you begin? Making the decisions, such as whether or not to receive HRT, all too often are excruciating.

Fortunately, your most reliable resource to smoothly navigate through the transitions of menopause is right between your ears, says Mary Jane Minkin, M.D., clinical professor of obstetrics and gynecology at Yale University School of Medicine and coauthor of *What Every Woman Needs to Know about Menopause*. The first thing to know is that a good treatment for one woman is not necessarily the ideal plan for you. You have the capability—and the responsibility to your long-term health and happiness—to carefully consider current medical information, create a self-care plan unique to your needs, and seek help if you need it.

Remind yourself through the journey that doctors have some answers, but certainly not all of them. In fact, half of the 925 family physicians interviewed for a study done at the University of Wisconsin Medical School in Madison incorrectly answered basic questions about menopause. In the enlightened 1960s, a leading hormone researcher proclaimed that the menopausal woman "suffers from a vapid, cowlike misery . . . she becomes the equivalent of a eunuch. "Hogwash," say the nation's top experts interviewed for this book.

"I certainly don't see menopause as a disease," says Jesse Hanley, M.D., a physician who specializes in women's health, medical director of Malibu Health and Rehabilitation in California, and coauthor of *What Your Doctor May Not Tell You about Premenopause*. "It is a natural life transition that can bring beauty, power, and purpose to a woman's life."

You owe it to yourself to explore the facts and dictate a self-care strategy, says Dr. Windstar. "Menopause is the ultimate time for women to start taking health into their own hands."

See Alternative Options, beginning on page 121, if you want to find medical practitioners who can help you develop deeper perceptions of your own physical, emotional, and even spiritual well-being. These holistic practitioners can also counsel you in nondrug hormone maintenance and other self-directed forms of management.

Your Self-Care Strategy

Dr. Nichols teaches this basic method of personal evaluation.

Draw a line down a sheet of paper. On the left side, write down all of your inherited risk factors, such as heart disease or stroke in your family, relatives with osteoporosis, and a mother or sisters who had early menopause. This is also where you write down symptoms that you can't live with— like excruciating hot flashes that don't respond to home remedies. The longer the left side (the uncontrollable risk factors and more severe symptoms) of the list, the more hormone therapy might be in your favor, she says.

On the right side, write down the risk factors that you *can* control, including your cholesterol levels and unhealthy lifestyle habits like smoking, a high-fat diet, and stress. Here's where you also list symptoms, like occasional hot flashes, which don't disrupt your life enough to warrant medication. After reading this book, include in this right-hand column things that you plan to do to resolve these issues, like taking the herb black cohosh to calm your hormones or taking a tai chi class to relieve anxiety.

The list accomplishes two tasks, says Dr. Nichols. It spells out what risks and symptoms you might be able to reduce on your own with lifestyle modifications rather than turning to medication. It also indicates what tests you might need for more information.

Determine whether you're up to date on bone-density tests and cholesterol readings, which vary from yearly to much less frequently according to a woman's health profile. Ask your doctor if you should be getting annual or biannual mammograms along with your annual Pap test. You should reevaluate this list as you get new test results or if your symptoms change.

If your risks or symptoms weigh out on the side of hormone replacement, it's important to know that your doctor has more methods to customize hormone therapy than she would have in previous generations. The American College of Obstetricians and Gynecologists reports that both temporary use of HRT and new combinations of hormones are becoming popular treatment options.

For instance, heavy menstrual bleeding might be resolved by reducing the amount of estrogen. Depression symptoms might call for a higher level of DHEA in the hormone lineup. And some doctors are prescribing natural progesterone (rather than the more widely used synthetic form) with standard estrogen for part of the month. "There is a certain percentage of women (15 to 20 percent of HRT users) who simply just don't feel any benefits while taking synthetic hormones but do much better with natural versions," says Dr. Minkin.

Forget the myth that you can't stop HRT once you start or that you have to take HRT forever, says Dr. Minkin. It's true that staying on long-range estrogen may offer protective benefits for osteoporosis and heart disease, but even temporary HRT can relieve specific symptoms during the hardest part of the transition, she points out.

No matter what you decide about HRT, if you follow the suggestions in this book for fine-tuning your lifestyle, you can achieve an easier, if not invigorating, journey through menopause. But good health is not just about eating more soy or finding time to work out. Your attitude matters tremendously.

According to studies at the University of Massachusetts and the University of Pittsburgh, women who predicted that they would have a difficult menopause did, in fact, suffer more negative emotional and physical symptoms than women who expected that it would go smoothly. So make a commitment to calming your spirit and challenging your mind, too. The advice in Managing Your Many Moods, beginning on page 69, can coach you through a positive voyage by using your experience as a time of personal discovery. It also offers so many nurturing ideas that you'll never need to visit a spa again.

Be open to trying a variety of home remedies on these pages to get the most complete care possible. You'll have more than 100 doctor-approved suggestions to prepare you for the next and, more often than not, best part of your life.

Eating for Your Future

"When your eating is under control, everything else feels more in control, too. Instead of eating for comfort and making everything worse, eat for health and energy to support positive change."

—Edith Howard Hogan, R.D., L.D., *nutrition counselor specializing in women's health and spokesperson for the American Dietetic Association in Washington, D.C.*

AVOID FLASH FOODS

Tea, coffee, and other hot or spicy foods and drinks can provoke the sweaty spells we all dread.

During menopause, your body struggles to control its internal thermostat. All too often, it fails. Toss in caffeine with its stimulating effects, and things get worse. Serve it up hot, and, if you're prone to hot flashes, you'd better head for the deep freeze.

"I tell my patients that hot coffee and hot tea are no-no's if they want to minimize hot flashes," says Mary Jane Minkin, M.D. Hot drinks add more warmth to your body, and this burst of heat can overload your erratic temperature mechanisms. Caffeine also relaxes your capillaries and allows more blood and heat to reach your skin, creating the unwelcome flush. Alcohol has a similar warming effect.

Spicy foods, too, can superstimulate more than just your tongue. Greatly limit your intake of whole peppercorns, crushed red pepper, and even freshly ground pepper, says Dr. Minkin. Steer clear of chiles in Southwestern, Mexican, Indian, and Chinese foods. Remember that the smaller the chile, the hotter it usually will be.

—Mary Jane Minkin, M.D., *is a clinical professor of obstetrics and gynecology at Yale University School of Medicine and coauthor of* What Every Woman Needs to Know about Menopause.

TREAT THIS GERM LIKE A GEM

Wheat germ is packed with so many nutrients that many researchers consider it the ultimate health food for menopausal women.

Wheat germ is a concentrated source of vitamin E and folate, both of which have been shown to protect against heart disease, says Densie Webb, R.D., Ph.D. "It's also packed with manganese, magnesium, phosphorus, and potassium—trace minerals recently shown to be critical for strong bones."

Wheat germ is a part of the wheat kernel, which, along with the fibrous bran coating, gets processed out to make white flour, so most women don't get very much of it. But you can add it back into your diet in a variety of ways. When you're baking muffins or quick breads, replace ½ cup of flour with wheat germ. In cookies, go up to 1 cup. You can also swirl it into smoothies, stir it into yogurt, or sprinkle it on cold cereal and salads.

At room temperature, wheat germ spoils quickly. So refrigerate it in a tightly sealed container. That way, it will stay fresh for up to 9 months, says Dr. Webb.

—Densie Webb, R.D., Ph.D., *is a nutritionist in Austin, Texas, and associate editor of* Environmental Nutrition *newsletter.*

WATER DOWN SYMPTOMS

Being even just a little dehydrated can trigger a range of menopause aggravations. So drink up.

Staying well-hydrated is vital for cooling down those hot flashes and fending off constipation, irritability, insomnia, and other symptoms of menopause, says Felicia Busch, R.D. Getting enough water also can help you feel more energetic and can even diminish skin dryness.

Here are a few solid ways to avoid dehydration and to drown out menopausal symptoms.

- Drink six to eight 8-ounce glasses of water daily. If you're active, especially in hot and humid weather, drink more.
- Cool water is absorbed more quickly into your body than warm water, says Busch. So chill your water bottle in a freezer for a few minutes before you head out to the golf course or tennis court. Your water is also more apt to stay cold until the end of your game.
- Plain water is fine, but if you prefer the flavor or carbonation of bottled water, that works just as well. Do whatever it takes to keep your tank full.
- Limit your consumption of cola, coffee, and other caffeinated drinks since they are diuretics, which move water out of your body.
- Think you're hungry? Have a glass of water first. Thirst often masquerades as hunger.

—Felicia Busch, R.D., *is the author of* The New Nutrition: From Antioxidants to Zucchini *and is based in St. Paul, Minnesota.*

COLOR YOUR LIFE
WITH CANCER PROTECTION

Women who eat lots of fruits and vegetables have the lowest rates of many kinds of tumors. Plus, research suggests that eating lots of high-fiber produce may protect against breast cancer.

Many postmenopausal women fear breast cancer—and with good reason. The older you get, the higher your risk of this dreaded diagnosis. One out of eight women experience breast cancer by age 80. But there's something that can protect you, and fortunately, it's right out back in your garden, says cancer researcher Cyndi Thomson, R.D., Ph.D.

Eat a minimum of seven servings of fruits and vegetables daily in all hues of the rainbow, she suggests. That's because carotenoids, the plant chemicals that create bright colors in fruits and vegetables, may help prevent cancer. So make it a habit to dine on blueberries, grapes, raisins, plums, dark green lettuce, spinach, kale, collards, carrots, strawberries, tomatoes, beets, and red, green, orange, and yellow peppers.

Try a new fruit or vegetable each week and learn new ways to prepare old favorites. You don't have to give up meat completely, just shift toward a more colorful plant-based diet. A good tool for expanding your produce menu is a vegetarian starter cookbook, such as *Vegetarian and More!* by Linda Rosensweig.

—Cyndi Thomson, R.D., Ph.D., *is a diet and breast cancer researcher at the University of Arizona in Tucson.*

PUT THE CRUNCH ON HEART DISEASE

Pecans, almonds, and other nuts can help slash your heart disease risk after menopause.

Nuts may be better than you may think they are cracked up to be. It's an injustice to their other health benefits if you shun them just because they contain fat. Eating just 1 ounce daily, about ¼ cup, can lower "bad" low-density lipoprotein (LDL) cholesterol levels, slightly raise "good" high-density lipoprotein (HDL) cholesterol levels, and lower triglyceride levels—a triple treat that protects against postmenopausal heart disease, says Kenneth I. Burke, R.D., Ph.D.

Walnuts, for instance, are the best land-based source of omega-3 fatty acids, the heart-protective oil found in salmon and other cold-water fish. Pecans, just like olives, are rich in oleic acid, another cardiovascular power broker. Almonds, too, are a bountiful source of heart-healthy natural vitamin E.

Just be sure to crunch with control. Each level measuring tablespoonful of these nuts packs about 50 calories, which can lead to weight gain and, in turn, overtax your heart. So measure your portions. Sprinkle a tablespoon of toasted walnuts on your hot or cold breakfast cereal, stir a tablespoon of sliced almonds into yogurt, or scatter 2 tablespoons of chopped pecans on a dinner salad, until you've reached your daily ¼-cup quota.

—Kenneth I. Burke, R.D., Ph.D., *is professor and associate chairperson of the department of nutrition and dietetics at Loma Linda University in California.*

BEFRIEND BROCCOLI

Cruciferous (cabbage family) vegetables are well-established cancer fighters. Now comes word that broccoli is also a potent ally in your fight against postmenopausal heart disease.

Like apples and onions, broccoli is a good source of flavonoids, a group of antioxidant compounds that scavenge free radicals before they can oxidize low-density lipoprotein (LDL) cholesterol. If oxidized, this bad cholesterol can glom onto your artery walls, increasing your heart attack risk.

Researchers at the University of Minnesota hailed broccoli after they analyzed the eating habits of 34,000 postmenopausal women. After 10 years, those women who ate the most flavonoid-laden foods had a 32 percent lower risk of dying from heart disease than those who ate the least of this nutrient. Of all the beneficial foods studied, broccoli demonstrated the most promise. "This is the only study done exclusively on postmenopausal women that looked at flavonoids," explains Laura Yochum, R.D., who was the lead researcher. "It suggests that getting plenty of foods rich in flavonoids, especially broccoli, can lower the heart disease risks that escalate after menopause."

One cup of cooked broccoli is also good source of heart-friendly fiber and folate, as well as vitamins A, C, and E. To get the most nutritional benefit, buy broccoli that is bright emerald green with small, tightly closed flower buds, she says.

—Laura Yochum, R.D., *is currently a senior health care analyst in Phoenix.*

GET HOOKED ON DEEP-SEA FISH

Eating certain fish can help keep your arteries clear and lower your risk of heart problems as you go through menopause.

As menopause kicks in and your estrogen level tumbles, your risk of heart disease shoots up. But adding fish such as salmon, turbot, haddock, and cod to your menu two or three times a week can help keep your cardiovascular system healthy, says Clare M. Hasler, Ph.D.

That's because these deep-water ocean fish have developed a kind of body fat—called omega-3—that stays pliable no matter how low the temperature goes. When you eat these omega-3's, they become part of your own cell membranes, which, in turn, become more supple, says Dr. Hasler. That means the walls of your arteries are more flexible and the platelets in your blood are more slippery, a combination that can lower your risk of blood clots. (A blood clot that gets stuck in the artery that supplies blood to your heart is what typically causes a heart attack.)

Eat your fish baked, broiled, steamed, poached, grilled, or even canned. But avoid frying it. That only adds heart-clogging saturated fat to your meal. When you're eating out, order grilled salmon, have anchovies on your Caesar salad, or go for a tuna sandwich.

—Clare M. Hasler, Ph.D., *is the executive director of the Functional Foods for Health program at the University of Illinois at Urbana–Champaign and Chicago.*

PORTION OUT BALANCE

In order to minimize menopausal weight gain, you must select the right balance of foods on your plate. The bottom line: Slice starches, dice fat, value vegetables!

Menopause slows down your metabolic rate. To compensate, you know that your best move is to limit fat consumption. "But the downside of cutting too much fat is that it leaves you hungry," says Jackie Newgent, R.D. Many people then make the mistake of taking gluttonous helpings of carbohydrates instead.

The key to success, says Newgent, is to practice just as much portion control with breads and pastas as with cheese and meat portions. If you're fond of a big plate full of food, load up on veggies and legumes. "It's just a matter of balance," she says. "Remember that less fat, fewer starches, and more vegetables will help you maintain your premenopausal waistline and ease the burden on your postmenopausal heart."

She offers this Confetti Veggie Couscous as a quick and delicious example of a balanced one-dish meal.

Confetti Veggie Couscous

1   tablespoon extra-virgin olive oil
3   large cloves garlic, minced
6   ounces water
1   can (14½ ounces) vegetable broth
1   cup chopped red bell peppers
1   cup chopped zucchini or yellow squash
½   cup shredded carrot

10 ounces whole wheat couscous
¼ cup chopped fresh oregano, basil, parsley,
or a mixture
Salt, to taste
Lemon juice

Add the oil to a large saucepan over medium heat. Add the garlic and cook for about 1 minute, being careful not to brown the garlic. Add the water, broth, peppers, zucchini or squash, and carrot. Bring just to a boil over high heat. Stir in the couscous and herbs. Cover and immediately remove from the heat. Let sit for 5 minutes. Fluff with a fork and add salt. Serve immediately or chilled with a squirt of fresh lemon juice.

Makes 6 servings
Per serving: 295 calories, 3 g fat

—Jackie Newgent, R.D., *is a spa cuisine instructor at Peter Kump's New York Cooking School.*

BE SOY SAVVY

Soy is loaded with estrogen-like plant substances, which in moderation may help replace your body's subsiding hormone reserves.

Women in Japan and China eat lots of soy foods. The same women also don't need hormone-replacement therapy (HRT) since they have few menopausal symptoms, not to mention low rates of breast cancer. Better yet, research suggests that plant hormones in soy called isoflavones are responsible for building bone, thus lowering the risk for osteoporosis, which normally soars in menopausal years. Studies show that another plant hormone in soy, genistein, shows promise in fighting cancerous tumors.

So can eating soy help you avoid menopausal problems, as it does for your sisters living in the Far East? The medical community is not sure. Researchers have a number of misgivings and unanswered questions about this ancient Asian wonder. "The truth is, the Asian women who avoid symptoms have been eating soy all of their lives and may be benefiting from other factors in their diets or lifestyle," says Walter Willett, M.D., Dr.P.H.

In fact, some studies suggest that adding excessive doses of plant estrogens, like those found in soy products, to your diet later in life may actually *increase* your cancer risk.

So what should you do about this promising but perplexing legume? Dr. Willett recommends incorporating soy into your diet within limits. One or two servings of soy foods daily may be enough to give your estrogen a little lift, especially if you forgo HRT (women on HRT shouldn't need any help). Try a cup of calcium-fortified vanilla soy milk on your cereal. Snack on roasted soy nuts from the health food store. Marinate sliced tofu and portobello mushrooms, then grill and toss the mixture in a pita pocket or into pasta.

—Walter Willett, M.D., Dr.P.H., *is professor of epidemiology and nutrition and chairperson of the department of nutrition at the Harvard School of Public Health.*

PLUCK SOY'S FLOUR POWER

While the jury is still out on soy's benefits for bones, hot flashes, and breast cancer, it is clear that enjoying soy foods daily can lower your total cholesterol level by about 10 percent.

After the onset of menopause, a woman's total and "bad" low-density lipoprotein (LDL) cholesterol levels are likely to rise, while her "good" high-density lipoprotein (HDL) cholesterol level wanes, probably because of a dwindling supply of estrogen. Soy, because of its estrogen-like properties, may help halt that trend. Soy flour is a concentrated soy protein, with about 20 grams per ½ cup. It takes about 25 grams per day to get soy's cholesterol-lowering effect, says Barbara Gollman, R.D. This is an amount considered safe even if you're at risk for breast cancer (in some studies, excessive soy consumption is associated with cancer risk).

Since soy flour lacks gluten—the elastic component in wheat flour that allows bread or muffins to capture air so they're light and fluffy—you can't completely replace white flour with soy flour in recipes. "Try replacing about one-fourth of the wheat flour with soy flour, and watch the cooking time," says Gollman. "The soy will make muffins moist and tender, but they will brown a little more quickly." As a general rule, nip 5 to 10 minutes off the baking time suggested in a regular recipe.

To get you started on your soy adventure, try a Chef Gollman favorite.

Cranberry-Almond Muffins

½   cup light and firm silken tofu
    Peel of 1 orange, grated

½ cup sugar
2 eggs, lightly beaten
2 tablespoons canola oil
¼ cup soy flour
1¼ cups unbleached all-purpose flour
1 teaspoon baking powder
¼ teaspoon baking soda
¼ teaspoon salt
⅓ cup unblanched almonds, finely chopped
½ cup dried cranberries, coarsely chopped

Blend the tofu in a small food processor or blender until it reaches the consistency of mayonnaise, or whip with a handheld blender. (Do not use an electric handheld mixer.) Be patient, this takes several minutes.

Preheat the oven to 375°F. Coat a muffin tin with cooking spray. Set aside.

In a small bowl, mix the orange peel with the sugar until the sugar is orange-colored. In a medium bowl, combine the eggs, oil, and tofu. Turn the sugar into the egg mixture. Beat with a wire whisk until smooth.

In a large mixing bowl, combine the soy flour, all-purpose flour, baking powder, baking soda, and salt. Stir well. Add the nuts and cranberries. Add the tofu mixture and stir quickly, until just blended. The batter will be lumpy.

Fill the muffin cups about three-quarters full. Bake for 15 minutes, or until golden and springy to the touch.

Makes 12

Per muffin: 166 calories, 6 g fat, 1 g saturated fat, 35 mg cholesterol

—Barbara Gollman, R.D., *coauthor of* The Phytopia Cookbook, *is a Dallas-based consulting dietitian, nutrition educator, and culinary arts expert.*

SPREAD ON BENECOL'S BENEFITS

If you're tired of the battle of butter versus margarine in your low-cholesterol campaign, try Benecol on your bread.

Benecol, a margarine-like spread available in most dairy cases, can help keep menopausal estrogen loss from pushing your cholesterol sky-high. More than 20 clinical studies have shown that as little as three Benecol servings daily can drop total cholesterol by 10 percent and the "bad" low-density lipoprotein (LDL) cholesterol by 14 percent.

Benecol is a combination of canola oil and a powerful plant compound that helps block the absorption of cholesterol in your digestive tract. Unlike some margarines, regular Benecol spread—but not the "light" version—can be used to bake or sauté.

"It tastes good, and it actually melts," says Nadine Pazder, R.D. Try it on air-popped popcorn, baked potatoes, bagels, toast, and cooked veggies, pasta, or rice. You can even use it to scramble up your egg substitute.

Benecol's convenient premeasured packets make it easy to get the dose just right. "It is more expensive than butter or margarine, but I tell my patients it costs less than open-heart surgery," says Pazder.

Although Benecol is not a drug, be sure to check with your physician before using this product if you are taking cholesterol-lowering medication or if you are allergic to soy products.

—Nadine Pazder, R.D., *is the outpatient dietitian at Morton Plant Hospital in Clearwater, Florida.*

SWEETEN YOUR CHOLESTEROL NUMBERS WITH ORANGES

*Help yourself to a little citrus sunshine.
It's a surprising weapon in the fight
against postmenopausal heart disease.*

Researchers have long known that eating less saturated fat will lower levels of low-density lipoprotein (LDL), the so-called bad cholesterol. But food wasn't thought to have any effect on "good" high-density lipoprotein (HDL) cholesterol.

So Elzbieta Kurowska, Ph.D., was surprised when a group of individuals she studied, including postmenopausal women (none on hormone-replacement therapy), had a 20 percent increase in HDL after drinking three 8-ounce glasses of orange juice daily. Oranges are packed with vitamin C, folate, and other nutrients that could have a positive impact on cholesterol. But further studies will be needed to confirm Dr. Kurowska's results and to pinpoint the precise mechanism.

Dr. Kurowska is not advocating that you drink three glasses of orange juice a day. That's simply far too many calories for just one food, she says. Not to mention that some women in this small preliminary study developed high triglycerides, another risk factor for heart disease.

She suggests that you drink one glass of orange juice daily if you are a menopausal woman. That way, you'll still probably increase your good cholesterol without causing your triglycerides to sneak upward.

—Elzbieta M. Kurowska, Ph.D., *is a nutrition researcher in the department of biochemistry at the University of Western Ontario in London, Canada.*

GIVE YOUR BONES A BREAK FROM OSTEOPOROSIS

Calcium helps slow bone loss after menopause. But to get enough each day, you must think beyond the obvious.

When menopause occurs, a woman can begin losing up to 7 percent of her bone mass annually. Over time, that loss can lead to osteoporosis, a bone-thinning disease known as the silent crippler of women.

Doctors recommend that women up to age 50 get 1,000 milligrams of calcium daily and those over age 50 consume 1,200 milligrams daily. A glass of milk or 1 cup of yogurt is an excellent start. Each contains 300 to 400 milligrams of calcium. But to get a full dose, you're probably going to have to make a few changes in your diet, says Sheah Rarback, R.D. Here are just few ways to enhance your calcium intake.

- Replace the nondairy creamer in your coffee with ¼ cup of fat-free milk to be 75 milligrams of calcium richer.
- Sprinkle an ounce of shredded low-fat cheese on your salad, and you get another 200 milligrams of calcium.
- Top 1 cup of steamed broccoli with a tablespoon of sesame seeds, and get a vegetarian bonanza worth 82 milligrams of calcium.
- Scatter 2 tablespoons of slivered almonds on your green beans and get a 50-milligram calcium bonus.
- Snap up beans. Most contain between 50 to 130 milligrams of calcium per cup.

—Sheah Rarback, R.D., *is an assistant professor at the University of Miami School of Medicine in Florida.*

GET HIP TO VITAMIN K

If you're trying to avoid fractures caused by menopause-related bone loss, maybe you're eating plenty of dairy foods already. But a lesser known security to your skeleton is to kick up your K intake.

One out of every two women in the United States has an osteoporotic fracture in her lifetime. Decades of chronic pain and disfigurement can follow all-too-common vertebral compression fractures. If the injury is to the hip, a woman's golden years are likely to be blackened by permanent disability or premature death. One-quarter of the people who survive hip fractures require long-term care. Needless to say, it's imperative to take this insidious disease seriously, particularly when estrogen decline at menopause increases its likelihood.

Research shows that middle-aged women who get the most vitamin K from food have the lowest rates of hip fracture. The minimum recommended level of vitamin K is 65 micrograms daily, but experts say that to really bolster bones, you may need almost twice as much—about 110 micrograms.

"Green vegetables are the best source of vitamin K, which activates osteocalcin, a protein that makes your bones stronger," says Liz Ward, R.D. Just one brussels sprout or ½ cup of broccoli, cabbage, spinach, kale, Swiss chard, or collard greens will do it. For variety, try 1 cup of cooked asparagus, green beans, or turnip greens, or ½ cup of raw cauliflower. Vitamin K is also found in soybean oil and egg yolks.

—Liz Ward, R.D., *is a nutritionist in Stoneham, Massachusetts, and coauthor of* Super Nutrition after 50.

YELL FOR YOGURT

Want a supercharged source of calcium to strengthen your menopausal bones? Put plain yogurt on the top of your shopping list.

If you really want to do something to protect your bones after menopause, yogurt is a plain and simple skeleton helper.

Plain yogurt packs a whopping 400 milligrams of calcium per cup and is more readily digested than milk, says JoAnn Hattner, R.D.

In fact, as we age and head toward menopause, many of us lose the ability to break down lactose, the sugar in milk, and end up with bloating, cramping, or diarrhea. Many women who can't handle milk, however, do just fine with yogurt, Hattner says. That's because in the yogurt-making process, friendly bacteria digest a lot of the lactose for us, making our job much easier.

Also, with age, many women experience mild gastrointestinal symptoms. "Live and active cultures in yogurt keep your intestinal tract healthier," says Hattner. And that's in contrast to the problems some women have with calcium supplements. "Among the women I counsel, some become constipated from calcium carbonate supplements, while others develop loose stools from calcium supplements that contain magnesium. I tell them they'll do better with low-fat or fat-free yogurt.

"In its natural state, plain yogurt is higher in calcium than sweetened varieties. You can sweeten it yourself with honey and get a bonus because honey seems to fight infection," says Hattner. You can also use yogurt as a condiment by dolloping it atop soups and mixing it with grated lime peel as an accompaniment for fruit.

Whip up this simple dip for vegetables.

Creamy Mustard Dip

 1 cup calcium-added, low-fat cottage cheese
 ½ cup fat-free plain yogurt
 ⅓ cup brown mustard
 1 teaspoon chopped fresh thyme
 2 teaspoon minced shallots
 1 teaspoon chopped fresh dill or ¼ teaspoon dried
 ½ teaspoon lemon juice

In a food processor or blender, whip the cottage cheese until smooth. Add the yogurt, mustard, thyme, shallots, dill, and lemon juice. Stir until blended.

Use as a dip for fresh vegetables or dried tomatoes.

Makes about 2 cups

Per 2 tablespoons: 1 g fat, 100 mg calcium

—JoAnn Hattner, R.D., *is a nutrition counselor in Palo Alto, California.*

"D"EVISE A SUPPLEMENT STRATEGY

Your postmenopausal body simply doesn't process vitamin D and other vital nutrients like it used to. It's best to reach for a booster.

No matter how much calcium you pack in, it's worthless to your bones if you don't get enough vitamin D. That's the vitamin you make when sunshine hits your skin. All your life you have made plenty, but now as your reproductive system winds down, your skin doesn't work quite as efficiently. Neither do your kidneys, and one of their jobs is to transform the vitamin D that your skin makes into a form that your bones can use.

In your premenopausal years, you needed 200 IU of vitamin D daily. After age 50, in order to maintain strong bones, you need twice as much vitamin D, about 400 IU, and three times as much after age 70, about 600 IU. And this is one case where food isn't much help, says Kathleen Zelman, R.D. Milk has about 100 IU per cup only because it is fortified with D, but yogurt and cheese provide none.

The form of vitamin D that is available in most supplements is well-absorbed, so you should be well-supplied if you take a multivitamin or a calcium supplement with added vitamin D.

—Kathleen Zelman, R.D., *is an Atlanta-based spokesperson for the American Dietetic Association.*

SAY CHEESE

After menopause, your teeth and gums are more vulnerable to decay. A cube of cheese, however, can keep your smile turned up.

The loss of estrogen that occurs during menopause affects all the cells in your body, including the gum tissue surrounding your teeth. As your gums recede, tooth roots, which are not protected by hard enamel, become exposed to cavity-causing bacteria. And to make matters worse, baked, starchy foods like pastries, pretzels, crackers, and cookies stick between your teeth, providing the bacteria and the acidic conditions that rot teeth. The good news is that chomping on a piece or two of cheese, such as aged Swiss, Cheddar, or Monterey Jack, every day may actually protect against cavities, says Mary P. Faine, R.D.

Dairy products, cheese in particular, contain a protein that prevents plaque from sticking to teeth, she says.

Brushing or drinking water after snacks will also help fend off cavities. And if you experience dry mouth, chew high-fiber foods, such as celery or carrots. They stimulate saliva flow, which protects your teeth. A cup of fat-free milk is good saliva substitute because it won't cause cavities and it helps provide the calcium you need to keep your jawbone strong and your teeth sturdy.

—Mary P. Faine, R.D., *is an associate professor of nutrition at the University of Washington in Seattle.*

CREAM HARMFUL FLAVOR AGENTS

Nonfattening flavor enhancers will not only spice up your meals but also help you break away from eating habits that can undermine your postmenopausal health.

Old family favorites may suddenly seem bland and joyless when you banish their fat-laden ingredients in order to lower your cholesterol and corral your postmenopausal heart disease risk. But there is life after sour cream and bacon bits. You can avoid dieting doldrums by flavoring up food in new ways that will tempt your tastebuds, protect your heart, and fight cancer, too.

Start by replacing butter with extra-virgin olive oil, suggests Jackie Newgent, R.D. The flavor is robust, so you don't need much. And for weight control, think teaspoons, not tablespoons. Olive oil supplies a heart-healthier kind of fat, but it's still high in calories.

Cook with plenty of onions and fresh garlic, too, says Newgent. They're rich in organosulfides, compounds that create their characteristic "fragrances" and protect against heart disease and cancer. For best flavor and least fat, learn to "sweat" your vegetables (see following recipe).

Experiment with different herbs. Newgent particularly recommends rosemary. "Its pine fragrance entices you to indulge in dishes even if they lack the familiar smack of saturated fat," she says. Rosemary is also packed with carnosol, an antioxidant that may prevent cancer.

One last trick: Replacing ground beef with beans will eliminate the saturated fat and load you up on antioxidants that can defend cells against cancer-causing agents, Newgent says.

The next time you think "spaghetti," skip the meatballs and try Newgent's Chickpea Pasta instead.

Chickpea Pasta

> 1 tablespoon extra-virgin olive oil
> 1 large onion, thinly sliced
> 2–3 cloves garlic, minced
> 1 can (20 ounces) chickpeas, with juice
> 1 can (16 ounces) chopped tomatoes, with juice
> 1 tablespoon chopped or crushed fresh rosemary
>   Salt and freshly ground pepper
>   Hot-pepper sauce
> 2 tablespoons freshly grated Parmesan cheese
>   (optional)

Heat the oil in a large saucepan over medium heat. Cover the pan with a tight-fitting lid and "sweat" the onion and garlic by allowing them to soften and slowly release their own water without browning. If they begin to brown, reduce the heat.

In a blender, puree half the chickpeas and half (or all) of the chickpea juice. Stir the pureed chickpeas, whole chickpeas, tomatoes (with juice), and rosemary into the onion-garlic mixture. Simmer, uncovered, stirring occasionally for about 20 minutes, or until the sauce thickens.

Season with the salt and pepper and hot-pepper sauce. Stir in the Parmesan, if using. Serve over your favorite pasta or couscous or as a sauce for baked or grilled chicken.

Makes 8 servings

Approximately ½ cup sauce with 1 cup cooked ziti: 275 calories, 4 g fat, 13% calories from fat

—Jackie Newgent, R.D., *is a spa cuisine instructor at Peter Kump's New York Cooking School.*

GO AGAINST THE GRAIN

Americans are virtually addicted to white flour, white rice, and white sugar. Perhaps refined foods may look and feel lighter. But in reality, it is the darker, whole grains that can keep you lighter— and keep you alive longer.

When the diets of 34,000 women ages 55 to 69 were analyzed by researchers at the University of Minnesota, those who had diets high in whole grains were 40 percent more likely to live longer. Women who ate at least one daily serving of whole grain had a substantially lower risk of cancer, cardiovascular disease, diabetes, and other diseases, than women who ate almost no whole grain. And there's more good news: The whole grain eaters were significantly slimmer than the refined-foods fans.

"Women who eat more fiber usually weigh less, making it a welcome ally in the battle against menopausal weight gain and heart disease. That may be because high-fiber foods tend to be low in calories, yet bulky and filling, and they take longer to digest than processed foods," says Christine Rosenbloom, R.D., Ph.D.

Although the processed food industry so often sneaks stay-slim fiber out of common foods, it's worth it to go against the grain to get the right grain. When the germ and hulls are removed to make white flour and white rice, for instance, they lose fiber, along with precious nutrients. Whole grains, on the other hand, tend to be more satisfying because of their fuller, more satisfying flavor as well as the chewier textures that you can really sink your teeth into.

Most women eat 12 to 14 grams of fiber daily. But actually, you need to eat twice that amount, particularly as you go through menopause, says Dr. Rosenbloom. A great habit to increase fiber is to do your own baking with whole flours and oat bran, and base lots of meals around brown rice and wild rice, bulgur wheat, and buckwheat (kasha).

When you do buy processed foods, let the numbers talk. A "high-fiber" food supplies 5 or more grams per serving, while a food labeled as "a good source of fiber" provides 2.5 to 4.9 grams per serving.

Look for multigrain or whole grain cereals and crackers and switch to whole wheat pasta, pita pockets, and tortillas. For a bigger fiber boost, smash up bran cereal and use it as a topping for casseroles, vegetables, fruit, even frozen yogurt. And don't pass by popcorn—it's truly a fiber-friendly snack.

—Christine Rosenbloom, R.D., Ph.D., *is an associate professor of nutrition at Georgia State University in Atlanta.*

IRON OUT DIETARY WRINKLES

After menopause, your body's iron requirements change. You'll need to adjust your intake to protect your heart—and your overall health.

As long as you were having regular menstrual periods, you lost precious iron, critical for carrying oxygen for energy. That's why you always needed more iron than your mate (15 milligrams daily to his 10 milligrams) to avoid iron deficiency anemia. But after menopause, your iron needs drop to about 8 milligrams daily.

You still need this mineral, but you must make your intake more moderate, insists Kathleen Zelman, R.D. Some researchers suspect that excess iron can damage the heart and other cells in the body.

To get the right age-adjusted iron dose, take a senior formula daily multivitamin that contains 4 milligrams of iron, she suggests. Get your remaining daily iron needs from food.

Iron from lean meat, chicken, and fish is absorbed better than the iron from plant sources like beans, bread, fruit, or vegetables. Animal protein also increases the absorption of iron from those plant sources. So add an ounce or two of chicken to your beans, have a dab of lean meat with your potatoes, or have a bit of fish with your pasta. "You'll get all the iron you need without overdoing it," says Zelman.

—Kathleen Zelman, R.D., *is an Atlanta-based spokesperson for the American Dietetic Association.*

DASH AWAY
FROM HIGH BLOOD PRESSURE

More than half of all women over age 55 have high blood pressure. But dietary changes can begin to tame this "silent killer" in as little as 14 days.

When women reach menopause, usually in their late forties or early fifties, they are more likely than men of the same age to develop hypertension, also known as high blood pressure. Untreated, high blood pressure can lead to heart disease or stroke. But there's plenty that you can do to slash your risk of hypertension at menopause. For starters, eat less salt, lose weight, and cut down on alcohol. But to really take a load off your cardiovascular system, consider adding a powerful new weapon to your hypertension-busting plan—the DASH diet.

When people tried the Dietary Approaches to Stop Hypertension (DASH) program in research centers around the country, the results were remarkable. Research shows that shifting from a typical American high-fat diet to an eating plan that's low in fat, high in fruits and vegetables, and rich in low-fat dairy products could lower blood pressure as much as medication can, and in just 2 weeks, says Lawrence J. Appel, M.D.

The diet is pretty un-American, since it includes about double the national average consumption of fruits, vegetables, and low-fat dairy products. But it's well-worth the effort if you can get your blood pressure down without drugs, Dr. Appel says.

For best results, try to stay as close as possible to the following food proportions used in the DASH diet. If you're taking medication for high blood pressure, don't stop without your doctor's permission.

- Grains and grain products: 7 to 8 servings daily
- Low-fat or fat-free dairy foods: 2 to 3 servings daily
- Fruits and vegetables: 8 to 10 servings daily
- Meat, poultry, or fish: 2 or fewer 3-ounce portions daily
- Nuts, seeds, and legumes: 4 to 5 servings per week
- Fats and oils: 2.5 teaspoons a day

—Lawrence J. Appel, M.D., *is an associate professor of medicine, epidemiology, and international health at the Johns Hopkins Medical Institutions in Baltimore.*

TAKE PSYLLIUM WITH SUPPER

A potent ingredient in many laxatives, psyllium also can thwart heart disease.

Throughout your childbearing years, estrogen kept cholesterol under control, providing natural protection against heart disease. But with menopause, estrogen dwindles, which allows cholesterol levels and your risk of heart disease to soar.

Psyllium, the ground husk of the plantain plant usually grown in India, may be one of your best weapons in the battle against postmenopausal heart disease, says Gail Frank, R.D., Dr.P.H. Like oat bran, psyllium is loaded with soluble fiber, a gummy substance that clings to digestive secretions called bile. As this fiber passes through your digestive tract, it traps bile, which normally helps your body absorb fat and cholesterol from food. Without bile, more cholesterol is excreted from your body.

Just a little psyllium is mighty potent: 1 tablespoon contains as much soluble fiber as 14 tablespoons of oat bran. So even if you're already eating a diet low in saturated fat and cholesterol, adding 4 level teaspoons daily of ground psyllium seed husk to drinks and foods may further reduce your cholesterol load.

But beware: You can't eat psyllium by itself. It soaks up water like a sponge in your digestive tract and could cause constipation. Instead, stir it into at least 8 ounces of juice or milk or add it to cookies or muffins in place of a few teaspoons of flour. Psyllium also works well in meat loaf because it helps soak up the juices.

Add psyllium to your diet gradually. Start with 1 teaspoon a day for about a week. Add another teaspoon each week until you reach 4 teaspoons a day. If you develop gas or bloating at some point, cut back to your previous dosage. If even 1 teaspoon triggers these symptoms, stick it out for a week—your body may adjust. If it doesn't, cut back to ½ teaspoon for a week, then gradually increase your dosage as previously described.

Be certain to get your daily requirement of at least eight 8-ounce glasses of water. Plenty of water helps psyllium do its job. In addition, fluids will cut down on gas, bloating, and other side effects, says Dr. Frank.

Psyllium is available at most health food stores. Check with your physician before using the supplement because it can alter the absorption of medication you may be taking. Also, don't take psyllium if you have a bowel obstruction.

—Gail Frank, R.D., Dr.P.H., *is a professor of nutrition at California State University at Long Beach.*

GRIND DOWN THE POUNDS

There's no question that stealth pounds
can sneak up after menopause. But you can
make them vanish with these dietary tricks.

Excess weight gain, particularly after menopause, increases your susceptibility to heart disease, cancer, high blood pressure, stroke, diabetes, and joint disease. What are the best long-term dietary solutions? Try these strategies suggested by Edith Howard Hogan, R.D., L.D.

• Eat breakfast. Too often, women think that eating fewer meals will help them lose weight. But menopause causes a 4 to 5 percent dip in a woman's metabolic rate. When you skip breakfast, your body fights back by lowering the rate of calorie burn even more, making it more difficult to lose weight.

• Graze your way through the day with three meals and three planned snacks. Skipping meals can magnify your menopausal symptoms.

• Choose "one-fisted" snacks. A piece of fresh fruit, a miniature box of raisins, a cup of yogurt, a little box of cereal, a snack pack of applesauce, or a pop-top can of tuna automatically limits your portions.

• Shrink your sweets. Bite-size chocolate bars, presliced brownies, or mini bagels will give you the taste you love with portion control. Just be sure to say no to seconds.

• Downsize your dishes. Use a salad plate instead of a dinner plate for meals, a cup instead of a bowl for soup, and a juice glass instead of a tumbler for beverages (unless it's water, which you want to load up on).

—Edith Howard Hogan, R.D., L.D., *is a nutrition counselor specializing in women's health and a spokesperson for the American Dietetic Association in Washington, D.C.*

Helping Yourself through Physical Changes

"Exercise is good for everything. Research shows that women who exercise regularly will be less aware of things that can bother them during menopause, especially hot flashes."

—Mona Shangold, M.D., *director of the Center for Women's Health and Sports Gynecology in Philadelphia*

MAKE A DASH FOR RELIEF

You can literally run away from a multitude of menopausal symptoms if you take the right steps.

Experts and enthusiasts alike report that a regular running program can neutralize hot flashes, mood swings, and other menopausal symptoms. Additionally, running is an exercise that helps maintain bone density at a time when women lose it rapidly. It also can reduce blood pressure and heart disease risk.

Karen Nichols, D.O., recommends a combination walk-jog-run program, which is modeled after her own fitness regimen, which she's followed for the last 30 years. She freely alternates between the three speeds, depending on how strong she feels.

An interval approach to running is a safe and effective way to get started, according to the American Council on Exercise. Beginners should walk 50 yards, then jog the next 50 yards, and repeat this interval 10 to 20 times for no more than 30 minutes every other day for the first month. Gradually increase your jogging intervals up to 2 or more miles. You can use some intervals to sprint as you become better conditioned and experienced, says Dr. Nichols.

As a beginner, stick to gentler running in your first month. Wear well-cushioned running shoes that you haven't worn longer than a year, and avoid uneven running surfaces.

—Karen Nichols, D.O., *is an osteopathic physician and director of Southwest Medical Associates in Mesa, Arizona, and an officer with the American Osteopathic Association.*

BALANCE YOUR HEALTH WITH A BALANCED WORKOUT SCHEDULE

Exercise can lift more than your aging buns and breasts. It is also proven to lift your spirits—and increase your chances of staying disease-free.

Doctors have long stressed the big picture, that exercise can keep heart disease, osteoporosis, and other high-risk diseases of postmenopausal years out of your future. The more immediate benefit is the deep satisfaction of looking good on the outside and feeling great on the inside, even when shifting hormone levels threaten to aggravate self-esteem, anxiety, and depression, says Helen Healy, N.D.

According to a recent review of research by the American Psychological Association, 5 weeks of mild to moderate exercise activities can alleviate depression and may bring relief to those with panic disorders. What kind of exercise reaps these results? Positive outcomes resulted from both aerobic (cardio activities like running and walking) and anaerobic (weight lifting) activities.

Aerobics and strength training actually increase your body's natural feel-good chemicals. Weight lifting is particularly uplifting because you quickly see results on your newly contoured body. Once on a program, some women find that they look and feel even better than when they were younger, says Dr. Healy.

In addition, balance and flexibility activities like yoga, dance, and tai chi will release tension from your body and help you avoid accidents and injury.

"A balanced exercise program is one of the best things to ensure a smooth menopause," says Dr. Healy. The key to winning peace of mind through movement is to develop a workout routine that incorporates aerobic, strength-training, and flexibility activities—and practice them consistently.

Dr. Healy recommends a plan that involves 30 to 40 minutes of aerobic exercise 3 days a week. There are countless options to choose from, so experiment to find activities that you really like. You can fill your week with activities like a Sunday morning hike, a Tuesday morning swim routine, and a Thursday kickboxing class. Or you could try a weekend inline skating outing and daily mall walking dates with friends.

To reap weight training's solid results, sign up at the local gym for an experienced training partner who can help you to stay motivated and teach you proper form. Or follow a free-weight instructional video at home three times a week. Make sure to supplement your aerobic and weight training with a stretching routine before and after you exercise.

—Helen Healy, N.D., *a naturopathic physician, is the director of the Wellspring Naturopathic Clinic in St. Paul, Minnesota.*

CARRY YOUR OWN WEIGHT

Qigong, an ancient healing art, offers weight-bearing exercises that help strengthen your body while soothing your spirit.

Weight-bearing exercise is invaluable for any woman hoping to prevent bone loss associated with the drop in estrogen during her postmenopausal years. Despite what it is called, you don't have to pump any iron to stimulate your bones to regenerate—other than the weight of your own form. An ancient discipline that efficiently stimulates the spine, hip, and lower-body bones, in particular, is the Chinese art of *qigong* (pronounced "chee-gong").

Your skeleton and muscles become stronger in subtle ways while you gracefully move through different series of qigong movements, but you're more likely to notice the way qigong melts away your anxiety and irritability. That's why Martha Howard, M.D., calls qigong a comprehensive workout for menopausal women. "It's very nurturing to your body and your mind," she says, "like getting a complete acupuncture treatment and a workout every time you do it."

A qigong teacher or an instructional video can teach you hundreds of postures and movements. But for starters, Dr. Howard recommends a basic qigong movement that she calls the wall squat.

"I recommend getting into the intent of qigong form, which is a state of loving compassion," says Dr. Howard. "For the wall squat, imagine that you are bringing in loving energy as you are going down. As you come up, you are giving away the loving energy."

1. Start by leaning your back against a wall or a door frame, with your heels about 1 foot away from the wall and your feet together.

2. Bend your knees and slowly lower your torso toward the floor as you keep the back of your head and your back flush against the wall or doorjamb. Keep your heels in contact with the ground.

3. Finish the squat at about a 90-degree bend of the knees, with your thighs parallel to the floor. Don't go any lower than 90 degrees, or you could harm your knees. If at any point your knees are strained, slowly rise back up.

4. Slowly move back to the starting position without locking your knees at the top of the movement. Repeat the squat several times.

—Martha Howard, M.D., *is a physician specializing in herbs and holistic medical treatments. She is the director of Wellness Associates of Chicago.*

GIVE YOURSELF A LIFT

A quick and simple hand-weight routine can tone flabby arms and breasts and prevent weight gain in troublesome places.

One potential fallout of the postmenopausal years is literally the falling-down of muscles, especially in the back of your arms and, unfortunately, your breasts. But weight training can bolster your confidence in your appearance.

Weight training also protects against a weak skeleton by stimulating your bones to regenerate. Best of all, since muscles demand extra fuel, your metabolism has to burn a lot of fat cells to maintain them, says Bob Goldman, M.D.

Before starting weight training (or any exercise program), consult your doctor. You may also want to seek out a personal trainer to help you develop a complete workout and to ensure that you do it properly. Here are some simple hand-weight moves to get you started.

You can use 1-, 2-, 3-, and 5-pound hand weights. For each exercise, choose a weight that is challenging but is light enough to allow you to comfortably do 12 repetitions of the exercise. On standing motions, be sure to bend your legs slightly so that you don't lock your knees, and don't lean forward or backward.

Overhead triceps extension. This movement pinpoints the dreaded flabbiness on the back of your upper arms and helps you perform any pushing motions in everyday life. Start by holding a weight with both hands above your head,

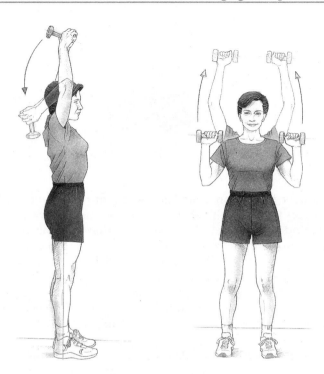

as shown on the left. Make sure that your upper arms and shoulders remain stationary as you slowly bend at the elbows and then slowly raise the weight.

Overhead press. Take a weight in each hand, and stand with your feet hip-width apart and your knees slightly bent, as shown on the right. Starting with your palms facing forward and your elbows bent so that each arm forms a V at your sides, slowly press the weights upward, until your arms are straight. Exhale each time you raise them and inhale as you slowly bring them back to the V position.

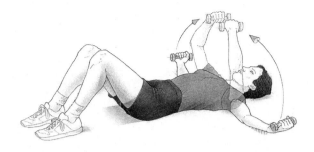

Chest fly. Lie on your back with your knees bent and your feet flat on the floor. Press your stomach toward your back and your back into the floor so that your pelvis tilts slightly upward. With your arms stretched out at your sides, hold a weight in each hand, palms up, slightly off the ground, with a slight bend to your elbows. As you exhale, press your weights up to each other while maintaining the arc in your arms, as shown. When the weights gently touch, inhale while slowly lowering your arms to the starting position.

—Bob Goldman, M.D., *is a sports medicine physician and chairperson of the American Academy of Anti-Aging Medicine in Chicago. He is also a senior fellow at Tufts University in Boston.*

SNEAK IN EXTRA STEPS

Boosting your physical activity doesn't have to mean going to the gym or revamping your schedule.

If you do only one thing to ensure happier and healthier menopausal years, it should be to get more exercise. Just about every expert recommends it for stabilizing your emotions while protecting against heart disease and osteoporosis. The problem is actually finding time to do it. That's why Yvonne S. Thornton, M.D., recommends sneaking it in.

"It's ideal if you are cycling and lifting weights at the gym each morning," says Dr. Thornton. But she understands that exercise doesn't always work into your schedule, and some days you're just not up to changing into spandex. Well, you don't always have to. You just have to be willing to put a little more oomph into your day's activities. "I tell patients to take the stairs and do their errands on foot whenever possible," she says.

You can make your housework more of a workout, too—hang out the laundry or use a push mower to cut the grass, for example. And when your chores are done, substitute more vigorous hobbies, like gardening and golf, for sedentary pastimes.

—Yvonne S. Thornton, M.D., *based in Morristown, New Jersey, is an associate clinical professor of obstetrics and gynecology at Columbia University College of Physicians and Surgeons in New York City and author of* Woman to Woman: A Leading Gynecologist Tells You All You Need to Know about Your Body and Your Health.

TWIST AND SHOUT

Dance is a great way to prevent bone loss and osteoporosis associated with menopause. Plus, it's a heck of a lot of fun.

No matter if you line dance, African dance, or waltz, dancing is one of best ways to keep yourself strong inside and out as you move beyond menopause, says Sadja Greenwood, M.D. Dance combines all three exercise elements—aerobic conditioning, muscle strengthening, and flexibility—that a woman needs to prevent osteoporosis, a bone-thinning disease.

In fact, one study in Vienna, a likely place if there ever was one to study ballroom dancing, showed that women with osteoporosis significantly improved bone density in their spines after 1 year of participating in a dance group 3 hours each week. Other studies support the same premise and also point to improved balance and coordination.

But you don't need a ballroom or advanced skills. You can simply put on some music at home and get moving, says Dr. Greenwood. If you do like cutting the rug with partners, public dances and classes are offered in most communities. Or you can find some live music and show your appreciation by twisting and shouting in the audience.

Check events slated for parks and recreation centers in the entertainment section of your local paper. And you can always get in step at a salsa, pop music, or oldies dance club.

—Sadja Greenwood, M.D., *is an assistant clinical professor at the University of California, San Francisco, and author of* Menopause, Naturally.

TAKE AN HERBAL CHILLER

Daily doses of black cohosh can cool hot flashes and may even electrify your love life.

Medical research suggests that black cohosh, a popular herbal remedy, contains estrogen-like substances that help relieve menopausal symptoms, especially hot flashes. Anecdotal reports suggest that black cohosh also can increase menopausal women's sex drives, says Kimberly Windstar, N.D.

But unlike conventional hormone-replacement therapy, black cohosh doesn't raise blood levels of estrogen. This makes the herb a particular boon for women who have experienced breast cancer, because it quells hot flashes without increasing the risk of recurrence, Dr. Windstar says.

Germany's Commission E (similar to the Food and Drug Administration), recommends a daily dose of 40 milligrams, taken for no more than 6 months. Some women find that one 40-milligram capsule is enough, says Dr. Windstar, while others might need to discuss increasing their dosages with their practitioners for best results. Because black cohosh is such a potent herb, it's best to consult your health care provider before taking it, she says, particularly if you are already on hormone-replacement therapy.

—Kimberly Windstar, N.D., *is a faculty member at the National College of Naturopathic Medicine and a naturopathic physician at New Health Horizons clinic, both in Portland, Oregon.*

BREATHE IN, ZONE OUT

Slower, fuller breathing can short-circuit middle-of-the-night hot flashes and get you back to sleep.

Hot flashes are never convenient, but they are particularly frustrating when they cut into your dream time. A soothing cup of herbal tea or a hot shower might help you relax enough so that you doze off again. But why get out of bed at three in the morning when a few deep breaths might do the trick?

We normally breathe in and out somewhere between 12 and 16 times per minute, says Toni Bark, M.D. She urges her patients who are awakened by hot flashes to slow their breathing down to about 10 times per minute. Often, doing that relaxes them enough so they can get back to sleep.

First, imagine your belly rising and falling with a slowed-down rhythm. Next, think of making your exhalations longer than your inhalations, and pausing between breaths. Start by inhaling for four counts, then holding for a count of five, and exhaling for a count of five. Work your way to several more counts, each time adding an additional count on the hold and exhalation.

—Toni Bark, M.D., *is a physician who specializes in homeopathy, a yoga instructor, and medical director of the Center for the Healing Arts in Glencoe, Illinois.*

GET TO THE ROOT
OF SLEEP PROBLEMS

Valerian is an an all-natural, nonaddictive remedy for insomnia.

Studies show that valerian has tranquilizing and sedative properties similar to the drug Valium. The added benefit is that it is nonaddictive, and it doesn't have the side effects, such as dizziness, that often can accompany prescription sleeping pills. All of this is good news for women who have difficulty drifting off to dreamland when menopause strikes.

To make a valerian tea, use 2 teaspoons of the chopped root per cup of boiling water. Steep for 10 to 15 minutes. Either add lemon and honey or mix it with juice since valerian has a strong taste. Drink a 1-cup portion of the tea before bed. Valerian is also available in capsule form. Take 200 to 1,000 milligrams (depending on the severity of your sleeplessness) ½ hour to 1 hour before your desired bedtime.

Don't use valerian with sleep-enhancing or mood-regulating medications. If you experience nervousness or heart palpitations, discontinue use.

When you purchase valerian from a health food store or herbal medicine supplier, be aware that valerian has a strong odor that often leads first-time users to suspect that they've gotten a bad batch. Don't worry, the pungent smell is normal.

—Varro Tyler, Ph.D., *is dean emeritus of Purdue University School of Pharmacy and Pharmacal Sciences in West Lafayette, Indiana, and author of* Tyler's Honest Herbal.

MAKE SCENTS OUT OF YOUR SYMPTOMS

Essential oils can provide a pleasant solution to a variety of discomforts and disruptions that menopause may bring.

One reason essential oils make you feel better is that they affect the endocrine system, says aromatherapy expert Victoria Edwards, R.N. Essential oils actually contain concentrations of plant estrogens similar to the ones in a woman's body that regulate her menstrual cycle. Essential oils can help balance the hormones that affect hot flashes, depression, insomnia, and vaginal dryness related to menopause.

Edwards has selected the following healing oils because they not only balance hormones but also have antispasmodic and relaxation effects. You can purchase the ingredients at health food stores or through an aromatherapy mail-order catalog. She offers several different recipes for particular symptoms of menopause.

For Tension, Hot Flashes, and General Discomfort

5   drops essential oil of lavender or rose geranium
2   drops essential oil of lavender sage (*Salvia lavandulifolia*)
5   drops essential oil of clary sage (*Salvia sclarea*)
1   ounce carrier oil

For Depression with Perimenopause

5   drops essential oil of cypress
5   drops essential oil of clary sage (*Salvia sclarea*)
2   drops essential oil of Roman chamomile
1   ounce carrier oil

For Insomnia

4 drops essential oil of sweet thyme
4 drops essential oil of rosemary
3 drops essential oil of sweet basil
4 drops essential oil of cypress
2 ounces carrier oil

For Lack of Vaginal Secretion

2 drops essential oil of Bulgarian or Turkish rose
2 drops essential oil of melissa
4 drops essential oil of geranium
1 ounce carrier oil

First, choose a carrier oil: either apricot, almond, grapeseed, or rosehip seed oil. Then mix your favorite carrier oil with the essential oil combinations in a sterile 60-milliliter glass bottle. Store your aromatherapy blend in the refrigerator with a tight lid.

Massage the oil into your skin, particularly over your heart, on the back of your neck, your shoulders, and your arms. After a bath or shower is a great time to do this, but you can use the oils any time you feel that you need it. You can also add these formulas (including carrier oil) to your bath, but be extremely careful or get help when getting out of the tub since it will be slippery.

Since essential oils do have medicinal qualities, please note the following precautions. Do not use cypress if you have high blood pressure, cancer, or breast or uterine fibroids. Do not use clary sage if you plan on drinking alcohol because it can exaggerate drunkenness and lethargy. Avoid rosemary if you have hypertension.

—Victoria Edwards, R.N., *is an aromatherapist, Jin jyutsu therapist, and an aromatherapy instructor for health care professionals in Fair Oaks, California.*

DIM THE BULBS

Lower the intensity of lighting an hour or so before you turn in. Your body chemistry will respond by making you dream-ready.

Your body produces the natural hormone melatonin, which regulates your body's sleep/wake cycle. Its production in the pineal gland is highest during nighttime hours, when light is in lowest supply. Dimming your lighting before bed can help melatonin put your body and brain to rest.

Melatonin supplements were touted a few years ago as a cure for jet lag and other sleep problems. But before you spend any money on them, try taking some simple measures yourself.

"Controlling light levels the hour before bed can encourage melatonin to make your body's natural transition from wakefulness to sleep, particularly when you are going through menopause," says Sadja Greenwood, M.D.

Here are Dr. Greenwood's bright ideas for getting your Zzzs.

- Turn off ceiling lights in the evening whenever feasible, and stick to desk or table lamps only. If you have dimmer switches, experiment with using the lowest levels comfortable.
- Put a low-watt bulb in your bedside lamp, just bright enough for you to adequately see the pages of your book or magazine (or consider a three-way bulb used at the lowest wattage at night).
- Install a reading light device that illuminates only your book page.

—Sadja Greenwood, M.D., *is an assistant clinical professor at the University of California, San Francisco, and author of* Menopause, Naturally.

SNUB OUT A PACK OF TROUBLE

Just one or two cigarettes per day can worsen hot flashes, sleep disturbances, dry skin, and mood swings.

At a time when hormone levels are already in flux, quitting smoking during menopause is essential. Nicotine can wreak havoc with your body's estrogen levels.

"Some women smoke in an attempt to self-treat the symptoms of menopause such as mood changes," says Mona Shangold, M.D. "They don't realize that smoking may be worsening their symptoms."

Even casual smokers who smoke one to five cigarettes per day—the people researchers refer to as chippers—are disrupting their hormone levels. In fact, studies show that women who smoke begin menopause about 2 years earlier than nonsmokers.

The sooner you snub out the habit, the better, Dr. Shangold says. Of course, it is best to quit in your twenties, but even women in their forties and fifties who quit tobacco can still tone down menopause symptoms by a few notches. There are many ways to quit—cold turkey, nicotine patches, or gums—and you may have to try several of them to snuff your urge to light up. But with perseverance, you can do it.

For strategies on quitting or to get support, contact the American Lung Association at (800) LUNG-USA.

—Mona Shangold, M.D., *is a gynecologist and director of the Center for Women's Health and Sports Gynecology in Philadelphia.*

SEEING IS RELIEVING

Visualization techniques can help control menstrual changes that affect three out of every four women just before menopause.

Heavy menstrual bleeding is a common complaint in the 3 to 5 years before menopause actually begins. Visualization can help you create a vivid image in your mind that can have a powerful physical impact on this problem.

To give it a try, take a few slow, deep breaths. As you begin to feel relaxed, close your eyes and allow your mind to create an image of your uterus. You might want to picture your uterus as having a large faucet. Use whatever concept works for you to get control over your menstruation. Now, imagine turning that faucet off. Watch as the flow slows to a trickle, then stops.

Practice your imagery several times a day as the time for your menstrual period approaches, suggests Tracy Gaudet, M.D. Although this process is called visualization, you can also use sound. Try to imagine a "drying up" sound or another sensation that is meaningful to you.

For some women, understanding the physiology of their bodies helps create potent images. In this case, know that heavy bleeding during perimenopause is caused when your uterine lining is thicker because you are not ovulating regularly. Looking at an illustration in a medical text or encyclopedia might enhance your visualization technique.

—Tracy Gaudet, M.D., *is executive director of the program in integrative medicine at the University of Arizona in Tucson.*

QUAFF KAVA KAVA'S KNOCKOUT PUNCH

This popular herb dissolves anxiety and dissipates bloating—two common symptoms that plague women in menopausal transition.

Although most modern scientific studies are still in preliminary stages, herbalists know that kava has long been brewed and served up in coconut bowls for relaxing social rituals. Kava is an ancient medicinal plant that has been part of the cultures of Pacific Ocean islands such as Fiji, Tahiti, Papua New Guinea, Samoa, and Hawaii for more than 3,000 years. For a menopausal woman under considerable stress, it can serve as a mild tranquilizer without being addictive or habit-forming.

You will find kava tea at health food stores and can take it according to package directions. For a soothing alternative, let kava tea brew in your bath with you (it will be absorbed through your skin).

Kava should not be used long term unless you're doing so under a physician's supervision. Do not mix it with alcohol, barbiturates, or antidepressant drugs because it can cause problems and side effects. It also worsens symptoms of Parkinson's disease. Do not take more than the recommended dosage on the package, and use caution when driving or operating equipment as this herb is a mild muscle relaxant.

—Varro Tyler, Ph.D., *is dean emeritus of the Purdue University School of Pharmacy and Pharmacal Sciences in West Lafayette, Indiana, and author of* Tyler's Honest Herbal.

OVERCOME INCONTINENCE WITH YOGA

Position yourself for stronger muscles and less stress with these simple exercises.

During menopause, a yoga practice can especially help you navigate the hormonal straits and fend off myriad symptoms. Incontinence is one issue helped by loosening up the spine and strengthening muscles in the trunk.

"A system like yoga provides for an entirely different way of treating incontinence than standard medical treatment, says Tracy Gaudet, M.D. Some of her patients with serious bladder problems were able to avoid surgery by using yoga to gain more control over their bodies.

The baby pose and the knee squeeze are two simple postures that she recommends not only to address incontinence but also to experience the overall stress-reducing effects of loosening up to spine. (For more information on the benefits of yoga, see page 127.)

Before beginning the baby pose, remove your glasses and shoes. Now sit on your heels with the tops of your feet flat on the floor. When your feet feel adjusted to the stretch, bring your torso toward your thighs by bending at the hip, until your forehead can be as flat as possible on the floor. If you are comfortable, move your elbows next to your sides with the backs of your hands facing the ground and enjoy the sensation of your back broadening, as shown.

If this full stretch is too much, you can lessen the intensity by crossing your arms in front of you and resting your head on them. Just breathe normally, keep your neck straight, and gently let go of any tension in your neck, spine,

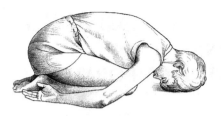

hips, and abdomen. Avoid this pose altogether if you have knee pain or high blood pressure.

Start the knee squeeze by lying flat on your back with your arms at your sides. Inhale as you raise your left knee to your chest. Wrap your arms around your knee and squeeze it into your chest.

Exhale and slowly relax, straightening your leg. Repeat with your right leg. Do three repetitions on each side, alternating sides, then rest a moment, breathing gently. Then try the same exercise, but lift both legs.

After a week or so of doing the double-knee squeeze, you may add the following step: After you squeeze your knees to your chest, lift your forehead as far as possible between your knees, then relax and breathe out. Go back to the easier versions if you have any pain.

—Tracy Gaudet, M.D., *is executive director of the program in integrative medicine at the University of Arizona in Tucson.*

MAKE THE MIND-BODY CONNECTION WITH HOMEOPATHY

Many menopausal frustrations can be remedied by learning to read your body's emotional and physical signs.

Homeopathy is system that uses dilutions of plant, mineral, and animal substances to stimulate the healing mechanisms of your body in very subtle ways. But the improvements that homeopathic medicine can bring to your well-being are far from subtle, says Janet Zand, O.M.D., L.Ac.

One reason why homeopathy can offer such powerful results is that the medicine is chosen on such a distinctly individual basis. To determine the correct remedy, you consider not only the obvious physical signs that indicate illness but also other more personal symptoms. In fact, emotions are just as important to your diagnosis as physical symptoms.

Choosing the appropriate remedy requires you to follow your instinct by matching even your quirky and minor signs with the best remedy profile. Check the following list to see if any sound as if they fit you, suggests Dr. Zand. If you don't have a close match, there are hundreds of other remedies to choose from by consulting a homeopathic medicine manual or discussing your symptoms with a practitioner.

Remedies can be purchased at health food stores or through a holistic practitioner.

- Aurum muriaticum is helpful if you are menopausal and find yourself in the throes of intense depression. Take one dose of Aurum muriaticum 30X or 15C three times daily for 3 days, as needed.
- Lachesis can restore your mind and body if you experience a combination of hot flashes, anxiety, and headaches. Take one dose of Lachesis 30X or 15C three times daily for 3 days, as needed.
- Natrum muriaticum is for dry skin and dry mucous membranes. If it is the correct remedy, you probably have cravings for salt. Take one dose of Natrum muriaticum 30X or 15C three times daily for 3 days, as needed.
- Choose Pulsatilla for menopause symptoms if you find yourself becoming upset and crying easily. Take one dose of Pulsatilla 30X or 15C three times daily for 3 days, as needed. Women who benefit the most from Pulsatilla usually have light complexions and are slight in figure.
- Sanguinaria is the remedy for you if you experience periodic occipital headaches (headaches that originate in the back of the head and travel over the eyes). You may also experience hot flashes and have hot hands and feet. Take one dose of Sanguinaria 30X or 15C two or three times daily for 3 days, as needed.
- Sepia is useful if you're feeling irritable. It usually benefits active, darkly complected women the most. Take one dose of Sepia 30X or 15C two or three times daily, as needed.

—Janet Zand, O.M.D., L.Ac., *is a naturopathic physician, a doctor of Oriental medicine, and a board and nationally certified acupuncturist practicing in Austin, Texas, and Santa Monica, California. She is also cofounder and formulator of Zand herbal formulas and author of* Smart Medicine for Healthier Living.

RUB OUT THE DROWSIES

Natural hormone creams can clamp down on fatigue and other menopausal symptoms without risky side effects.

When your hormones are on target, estrogen floods your body during the first half of your menstrual cycle. Then as you approach ovulation, progesterone takes center stage. It's a wonderful balancing act that worked well for years. But when menopause arrives, these hormones get out of synchronization. As a result, you may feel overwhelmingly exhausted.

Add in water retention, weight gain, irritability, headaches, and insomnia, and you're facing a rather bumpy ride through menopause.

The likely cause of this cluster of symptoms is too much estrogen and not enough progesterone, says Jesse Hanley, M.D. To relieve symptoms, doctors often prescribe synthetic progesterone, called progestins, but the medication can bring on another set of symptoms, which can include bloating, mood swings, breast tenderness, and irritability. Dr. Hanley recommends a nonprescription, plant-based progesterone cream as an effective and less invasive way to even out the estrogen-progesterone balance in your body.

Certain agents in yams and soybeans have been found to act like female hormones. In a topical cream, they can provide a natural alternative to synthetic hormones.

If you are over 40 and premenopausal, start using the cream now, Dr. Hanley urges. It will help nip many menopausal symptoms before they get out of hand. It can also help with hot flashes and vaginal dryness for any woman going through menopause. The cream is particularly beneficial for women who are prone to premenstrual syndrome, fibroids, or weight gain.

Rub ¼ teaspoon once or twice daily anywhere on the skin, Dr. Hanley suggests. Many women find it helpful to massage the cream into the skin near trouble spots, such as the breasts for cysts or the tummy for uterine fibroids (once you have them checked out and know they are benign, that is). Some of her patients have felt better in 1 month's cycle. If you have some spotting during your first cycle after you start using the cream, don't worry. It's normal.

The quality of natural plant-based progesterone creams can vary, so consult a qualified health professional to help you determine which product to choose. During menopause, discuss the use of the cream with your doctor to be sure that it fits into your overall treatment plan.

> **—Jesse Hanley, M.D.,** *a physician who specializes in women's health, is the medical director of Malibu Health and Rehabilitation in California and coauthor of* What Your Doctor May Not Tell You about Premenopause.

DEVELOP HABITS THAT HELP DRY SKIN

In menopausal years and beyond, you're going to need to take special care to keep your radiant exterior.

Pundits who refer to menopause as reverse puberty aren't kidding. When we were teens, the glands that produce a protective layer of oils in our skin were in overdrive, causing many a pimple-doomed date. But as we age, once-dreaded body oil is pined for, particularly by women who know that parched skin shows more wrinkles and is prone to itching and chafing.

These simple changes can make a moisturizing difference in protecting your skin from aging.

• Lower your thermostat. Dry skin is most problematic during winter because of dry air caused by indoor heat sources and frigid temperatures outdoors. Keeping your home thermostat below 70°F will help retain moisture in the air.

• Use a humidifier during cold-weather months when moisture is a commodity.

• Bathe and shower less frequently when temperatures are colder and the air is dry. When you do bathe, opt for quick showers rather than lingering baths. Use warm water rather than hot. Hot water can strip away the thin moisturizing layer on your skin.

• Use ointments made with camphor and menthol in times of severe dry skin. These moisturizers, such as Lac-Hydrin and Aquaphor, work best if they are applied when your skin is damp so the moisture gets "locked" into the skin. Just don't use camphor products at the same time as homeopathic remedies.

• Stay hydrated from the inside out by drinking eight 8-ounce glasses of water a day.

—Doron Nassimiha, M.D., *is a staff physician in the department of geriatrics and adult development at the Mount Sinai School of Medicine of New York University in New York City.*

Managing Your Many Moods

"Instead of focusing on what you might perceive as negative about menopause, you can say, 'Now is the time to take better care of myself, eat more healthfully, get enough sleep, and get rid of what is toxic in my life.'"

—David Simon, M.D., *medical director of the Chopra Center for Well Being in La Jolla, California, and author of* Vital Energy

AGE GRACEFULLY

*Is your attitude about growing older fair,
or is it ruled by society's stereotypes?*

It's no wonder so many menopausal women get depressed, living in the context of an 'ageist' culture, which assumes that growing older is an inevitable decline into incapacity, fatigue, and despondency, says Alice D. Domar, Ph.D.

"Certain changes do typically occur at midlife: It can be harder to lose weight, libido fluctuates, and social and family roles may shift. But none of these transitions should ever be interpreted to suggest that menopausal women cannot feel attractive, be fully sexual, come into their creativity, develop careers, or redefine relations with loved ones in ways that are profoundly gratifying," says Dr. Domar.

"Chances are, your distorted ideas about aging come from someone else's fear or stereotype. In other words, if your mind is a bus, who is driving it? Is it your boss? Your mother-in-law? Your father? A guy who broke up with you years ago? The media? For people who have negative beliefs running around their heads," says Dr. Domar, "the usual answer to 'who is driving your bus' is anyone but themselves."

Have the courage to question the origins of your negative impressions about menopausal and postmenopausal years. Then you can take the wheel and follow your self-guided directions on the road of maturity that lead to peace of mind and vitality.

—Alice D. Domar, Ph.D., *directs the women's health programs for the division of behavioral medicine at Harvard Medical School. She is an assistant professor of medicine at Harvard Medical School, a staff psychologist at the Beth Israel Deaconess Medical Center, and coauthor of* Self-Nurture.

CLIMB A MOUNTAIN OF CONFIDENCE

The transitional time of menopause offers us a great opportunity to follow our heart's desire, no matter how different it is from our present lifestyle. But first, we have to learn how to overcome the fears that may block us.

Sometimes called the change of life, menopause is an opportunity to experience more than just physical changes. It can be a turning point, where you change whatever you need to in order to get what you truly want out of life, says Susan Jeffers, Ph.D.

In terms of becoming the best you can be, it is important that you keep expanding your comfort zone to encompass more of the richness that life has to offer. With each risk taken, the boundaries of your life broaden and your confidence grows, so you are better able to push yourself through your fears, she says.

Dr. Jeffers offers these steps to making your change of life truly liberating.

1. Think of 14 risks you would like to take over the next 2 weeks, one a day, and list them on a sheet of paper. Include risks from different areas of your life, such as the following examples: career (making a cold sales call), relationships (asking someone for a date), independence (learning to drive), health (starting an exercise program), and creativity (taking up a new hobby). These may seem like big risks to you now. Don't worry. Start as small as you

wish. As you continue to take a risk a day, soon all risks will seem more manageable, says Dr. Jeffers.

2. Each evening, pick the risk you intend to take the following day. If you are feeling particularly brave, you may want to take more than one. Or you may find yourself thinking of a new risk that isn't on your list. That counts—just add it on.

3. Schedule your risk of the day on the calendar as you would a doctor's appointment.

4. After you've completed a risk, say to yourself, "Yes, I did it! What's my next risk?" You'll find that each risk you complete makes you willing to expand further, and taking risks gets easier as time goes by. Remember, action builds confidence.

5. If you're feeling hesitant about taking a particular risk, repeat the following affirmation over and over again: "Whatever happens, I'll handle it." After several days of this affirmation, try to take that risk again. If you are still unable to do so, just set it aside. Don't beat yourself up, but continue to recite the affirmation while you tackle other risks. "You will grow more each day as you build a mountain of confidence from which you draw strength," says Dr. Jeffers.

—Susan Jeffers, Ph.D., *is a doctor of psychology in Los Angeles and is the author of many best-selling books, including* Feel the Fear and Do It Anyway.

MAKE MENOPAUSE MEANINGFUL

In order to make menopause a healthy growth experience, take the time to really challenge yourself.

You have spent a lifetime dedicated to furthering your career, fostering a family, or both. But have you really invested in your most personal growth as much as you would like? Menopause is a rite of passage; make it meaningful, says Peggy Elam, Ph.D. Take inventory of your deepest desires, and consider ways to develop your interests. Use this life stage of entering new maturity to take on challenges that may be long postponed.

Dr. Elam offers these tips on making midlife a time of growth.

• Engage in a creative act every day. It can be freshly arranging your martini glass collection, cooking a different ethnic food each night of the week, or making your own Valentine's Day cards. If you're the type who needs structured discipline, sign up for a class to learn, for example, how to play the harp, grow herbs, or hang glide. If you *really* need encouragement, establish a creative partnership. "I have heard of two women who take turns sending each other postcards with a poem the sender wrote and a new topic for the next poem for the other to write," Dr. Elam says.

• Take the spotlight. You've had years to accumulate knowledge and wisdom. Let your confidence in knowing something show. Attend town meetings and express your views on the new zoning proposal. If they don't listen to you, run for the board. Serve as a tour guide at a local arboretum or historic area. Whether astute or quirky, celebrate your unique skills by teaching—offer a beginners' computer class at your town senior center, an egg-blowing workshop at church, a community discussion of Yiddish phrases, or a "Plumbing 101 for Women" class at a local night school.

• Lighten your load. Really contemplate what is and isn't working for you in your life, and then do some housecleaning—literally. Cleaning out drawers and closets not only is a practical way to manage the chaos, but it also can be a personal ritual to throw out reminders of old relationships and habits. Tell yourself while you are on your clutter rampages that you are moving out the old to create "space" for new, liberating experiences.

• Surround yourself with images and thoughts of menopausal and postmenopausal women who are vibrant and engaged in life and whose strength and wisdom you admire. Hang photos or pictures of those people and perhaps a quote from each one where you can see them every day. Now place a picture of yourself next to your heroines so that you are on an equal plane.

—Peggy Elam, Ph.D., *is a clinical psychologist and psychotherapist in Nashville.*

WRITE OFF SELF-CRITICISM

*The best way to challenge self-defeating
thoughts is to try writing down the
logic—or lack of it—behind them.*

In order for negative attitudes to be erased, you must un-
cover their messages, which may sound and seem true
until you really put them to the test of reason, says psychologist Alice D. Domar, Ph.D.

Here is a sampling of the negative thoughts that she
hears repeatedly from her menopausal patients.

- "I'll never feel attractive again."
- "My husband (or partner) does not want me anymore."
- "In terms of my career, it's downhill from here."
- "It's too late for me to realize my creative self."
- "My sex drive has declined, and it will only decline
further."
- "My children don't need me anymore."
- "I've gained weight, and I can't get it off."
- "I'm useless to my family and society."

You will be surprised at how responding to the questions
in the following test of logic can help you quickly overcome
these negative thoughts.

1. Where did I learn this thought?
2. Is this thought logical?
3. Is this thought true and fair?
4. How does this thought contribute to my stress?

Start by writing down the four responses to all the beliefs above that you feel relate to you. If you benefit, you can
make this an ongoing process by keeping a "diary of distor-

tions," in which you write down your automatic negative thoughts every day, always putting them to the logic test.

Just writing down the negative thought has therapeutic value. "It's a relief when you can say to yourself, 'There it is, the cause of so much suffering,'" says Dr. Domar. Better yet, once you are liberated from your distortions, your mind is free to restructure unjustified self-criticism into well-deserved self-respect.

—Alice D. Domar, Ph.D., *directs the women's health programs for the division of behavioral medicine at Harvard Medical School. She is an assistant professor of medicine at Harvard Medical School, a staff psychologist at the Beth Israel Deaconess Medical Center, and coauthor of* Self-Nurture.

SOUND AWAY MENOPAUSAL STRESS

A mind-body technique called toning can help bring back harmony if you're experiencing menopausal mood swings and other symptoms.

The use of the voice is a built-in tool that releases emotional tension from your body," says sound researcher Don Campbell. "A daily practice of toning, which is making a sound with an elongated vowel for an extended period, can improve your overall state of mind."

Toning is a great help for releasing and harmonizing your emotions during and following menopause because it moves your emotions through your body so that you do not feel pent up, vulnerable, or ready to explode, he explains. When your body responds to the vibration you are creating, even your hormone levels even out.

Campbell tells of a student who claims that she benefited so greatly from a toning practice that she could get off hormone replacement and say goodbye to her hot flashes.

Following is a brief outline of Don Campbell's 5-Day Toning Class. Do each exercise for about 5 minutes, holding the tone continually with natural breaths in between. If you enjoy the experience, repeat it whenever you need some relaxation or reviving.

Day 1—Hum: Sit comfortably, close your eyes, and hum—not a melody, but a pitch that feels comfortable. Relax your jaw and feel the energy of the hum warming up and energizing your entire body.

Day 2—Ah Sound: The *Ah* sound immediately evokes a

relaxation response. Whenever you feel a great deal of stress and tension, relax your jaw and make a quiet *Ah*. In your office or other places where toning may disturb others, you can simply close your eyes, breathe out, and think the *Ah*.

Day 3—*Ee* Sound: The *Ee* can awaken your mind and body, functioning as a kind of sonic caffeine. When you feel drowsy while driving or are sluggish in the afternoon, making a high *Ee* sound will stimulate your brain and keep you alert. The *Ee* tone is also good for releasing tension. Just don't practice it if you have a headache, or else the increased activity in your brain may make it worse.

Day 4—*Oh* Sound: The *Oh* tone is a great tool for an instant tune-up. Your body responds to the *Oh* by normalizing your skin temperature, breathing, and heart rate as well as releasing muscle tension and increasing brain waves.

Day 5—Experimental Singing: Start at the lowest part of your voice and let it glide upward, like a very slow elevator. Make vowel sounds that are relaxing and that arise effortlessly from your jaw or throat. Allow your voice to resonate throughout your body. Now explore the ways in which you can massage parts of your skull, throat, and chest with long vowel sounds.

> **—Don Campbell** *is the author of numerous books and instructional tapes on sound and health, including the best-selling* The Mozart Effect. *Drawing from work with prominent musicians, therapists, and mind-body researchers, Campbell founded the Institute for Music, Health, and Education in Boulder, Colorado.*

ALLEVIATE ANXIETY WITH ACUPRESSURE

A few minutes of acupressure, the fine art of finger pressure, can help ease your body and mind.

If you are experiencing feelings of anxiety as you approach midlife, or if you find yourself generally feeling stressed-out, acupressure can provide you with calming relief, says Oriental medicine doctor David Nickel, O.M.D., L.Ac.

How does it work? A practitioner could give you a lengthy explanation about how acupressure restores complex, energetic pathways in your body. But in Western terms, pressing your fingers or knuckles in the right places improves circulation throughout your body, including your brain. The resulting flood of minerals, enzymes, oxygen, and pleasure chemicals brings relief from muscular and emotional tension.

Dr. Nickel offers these acupressure points for anxiety. Practice each exercise on both the right and left sides of your body for maximum results.

With the tip of your forefinger, locate the neurogate acupressure point at the base of the upper ear triangle, as shown. Breathe so that you exhale through your mouth as you apply pressure and inhale through your nose as you ease pressure. Use a deep, relaxed breathing style. Con-

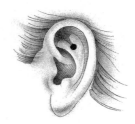

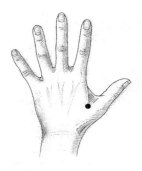

tinue this pressure-on, pressure-off cycle for 1 minute.

Next, feel for a tender spot in the web between your thumb and index finger. Hold the web of either hand between the thumb and index finger of your other hand, with the thumb on top and the index finger underneath. Squeeze gently but firmly for 5 to 10 seconds while exhaling through your mouth. Release the squeeze and gently inhale through your nose. Continue this pressure-on, pressure-off cycle for 1 minute.

—David Nickel, O.M.D., L.Ac., *is a doctor of Oriental medicine and a licensed acupuncturist in Santa Monica, California.*

STAND UP FOR YOURSELF

Using yoga to improve posture may bring multiple mind-body benefits to menopausal women.

Self-confidence is a by-product of good posture. By standing correctly, you increase your body's supply of oxygen and improve your blood circulation, which alone can bring a heightened sense of well-being. You may also become more mentally focused and emotionally grounded when you stand tall and sure, says yoga instructor Linda Rado.

On the other hand, poor posture may compress your internal organs, impeding circulation and digestion. If you're feeling lethargic or insecure, slumping in your chair or on your feet will only enhance the effect.

Rado offers the yoga exercise, mountain pose (also known as Tadasana), so you can feel for yourself what a difference it makes to stand well.

"Enjoy the simple and profound feeling of empowerment from the mountain pose. The mountain pose is especially pleasing to practice anytime you are waiting in line. Try it next time, and notice the effect," she says.

Here's how to practice the mountain pose.

• Stand with your feet turned slightly inward, the big toe joints about 1 inch apart and the heels slightly farther apart (about 2 inches). Allow your arms to hang naturally at your sides.

• Bring your chin back a bit, lift the crown of your head upward, and lengthen the back of your neck so that, from the side, your ears are in alignment with your shoulders. Your forehead will be parallel with the wall in front of you.

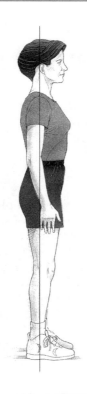

• Allow your face to soften and relax.

• Broaden your chest from the center, almost as if it were "blooming" like a flower. Don't stick your ribs out. The bottom ribs move down *slightly* toward your hipbones.

• Place your pelvis in a neutral position. To find this position, imagine that you have a long tail, and place the tail on the floor between your heels. This will align the pelvis nicely.

• Spread your toes and stand firmly on your feet. Keep your legs straight without gripping your thighs and move your thighbones back slightly.

• Breathe normally. Close your eyes for a few moments and pause. Become still. Then open your eyes slowly.

—Linda Rado, R.Y.T., *is a professional yoga teacher, yoga therapist, and co-owner of The Studio, a yoga center in West Reading, Pennsylvania. Certified in three schools of yoga, she continues advanced studies at Master Yoga Academy in La Jolla, California.*

LIGHTEN MENOPAUSAL MOODS WITH LAUGHTER

Dwindling fertility hormones may be an unstoppable fact of life, but you can certainly boost your "feel-good" hormones.

Research shows that laughing produces beneficial physiological effects because it reduces the release of stress hormones from the adrenal gland, while increasing the production of endorphins, the body's natural feel-good hormones. "Humor can reduce anxiety, soften anger, lighten depression, and raise your tolerance for pain. In all seriousness, laughter is beneficial for your body, mind, and soul, particularly when you are going through difficult times," says David Simon, M.D.

Here are some ideas for entertaining your playful spirit.

• Make your own compilation videos of film clips and television episodes that make you laugh. That way, you'll have them on hand when you need to lighten up. You can also rent or buy a compilation tape like *Saturday Night Live* reruns and watch bits of it every night.

• Stock up on silliness. Keep joke books and comics that are laugh-out-loud funny by your bed, in the bathroom, on the refrigerator—anywhere that you can always see them.

• Take a stand-up artist for a ride. Get cassettes and compact discs of comedians that you can listen to in your car so that long drives find you jolly.

• Humor your inner clown. Go to a photo booth with a friend and take whimsical pictures. Or cut and paste you and your family's, friends', or coworkers' photos onto pictures you find in magazines. Also, make a different goofy face in the mirror with each bathroom visit throughout the day. And get yourself a pair of Groucho glasses or a silly wig as a reminder to not take yourself too seriously.

- Sign up for a free joke-a-day service on the Internet via e-mail. Just type "joke" on your Web browser, or try logging on to Web sites such as www.humorproject.com, www.aath.org, and www.joke-of-the-day.com.

- Catch the bug. Laughter is not only the best medicine, it's contagious, too! When you read a jocund anecdote, quote, or cartoon, post it on your front door or someplace where you will be able to enjoy others enjoying it, too.

- See the comical side of the change. Read a funny book about menopause like *The Noisy Passage* by Marie Evans and Ann Shakeshaft.

- Instead of the typical dinner and a movie, why not take dates to comedy clubs or social clubs that feature a comic for the night's entertainment?

- Don't be a party pooper. When you host or attend parties, suggest funny-bone-tickling interactive games like Pictionary, Cranium, Taboo, Guesstures, and Balderdash. Or play poker for a ridiculous stake like gummy bears.

—David Simon, M.D., *is medical director of the Chopra Center for Well Being in La Jolla, California, and author of* Vital Energy.

SEND YOUR TROUBLES OUT TO SEA

Mental imagery can prevent menopausal symptoms from putting a damper on your plans to shine.

Mental imagery is a quick and natural method to take control of negative sensations that might arise during menopause. Gerald Epstein, M.D., offers this classic technique to relieve anxiety, depression, or hot flashes.

Sit in a comfortable chair, preferably with a high back and armrests for support. Place your arms on the armrests and your feet flat on the floor. Close your eyes and breathe out and then in three times slowly. Imagine yourself on a beach.

As you are looking at the sky far over the ocean, it begins to cloud over. You are hearing claps of thunder and seeing streaks of lightning as the storm gets closer and closer, gradually intensifying. Then, instead of letting loose, the dark clouds roll behind you, and the sounds stop and the flashes cease. Looking out into the ocean, you see the sun come up in the sky and know that your symptoms have passed.

To stay in control of your emotions, do this imagery exercise three times a day at the same time each day. You can also practice the imagery exercise at the first sign of a symptom and continue until the difficulty is over.

—Gerald Epstein, M.D., *is a mind-body physician in New York City and a pioneer in the uses of mental imagery. He is also director of the American Institute for Mental Imagery and author of* Healing Visualizations.

WELCOME SUPPORT

Nourish emotional and physical improvements among other women experiencing menopause.

Much research has shown that a support group can be an essential element in enhancing both mental and physical health. In a 10-year Stanford University study of women with advanced stages of breast cancer, researchers found that the women who were in a support group lived twice as long as those who were not in a support group.

"The group process offers wonderful energy to support change," says counselor Louise Hay. A menopause support group can be a focused opportunity for women to share the process of identifying their limiting beliefs, practice different techniques to improve their lives, and celebrate successes.

Just don't use your group to sit around and play "ain't it awful . . ." It does no good to support old patterns and to see who has the worst life this week. Instead, use the group as a stepping-stone in your growth process, says Hay.

To locate a women's support group in your area, check the local newspaper under "community meetings and services." You can also contact the National Self-Help Clearinghouse at 365 5th Avenue, Suite 3300, New York, NY 10016. Another option is to jump online for a menopausal women's chat room.

—Louise Hay *leads metaphysical study groups and empowerment workshops and is the author of numerous self-growth books, including* Empowering Women: Every Woman's Guide to Successful Living.

VOLUNTEER TO GROW

Volunteering may present itself as self-sacrificing and noble, which it is. But even more so, it can be one of life's most richly indulgent activities.

Your motivation may be out of respect for humanity, but the bonus is that in the end, volunteering truly heightens your own sense of self-worth. Get involved in making a difference in someone's life. In the process, you will discover your talents and abilities and explore interests and skills you never may have had a chance to explore. It is also a great way to meet new people that share similar interests, says psychotherapist Michelle Wheat Dugan.

"There are two reasons I personally volunteer," says Dugan. "One is that I feel that if each person doesn't take some individual responsibility to step out of their comfort zone and give something, the world is in for a rude awakening. But more and more, I am connecting with volunteer work on a spiritual level. In fact, I never feel depleted by giving. I feel energized by it."

A study called "The Woman's Roles and Well-Being Project" observed the lifestyles of 427 wives and mothers from upstate New York for 30 years. An exciting outcome: Women who belonged to volunteer organizations had significantly lower rates of illness, better mental health, and greater longevity.

What could be a better way to use retirement leisure time or make one of your free nights a week meaningful? There are many volunteer opportunities everywhere you go. Animal shelters, women's clinics, museums, children's sporting events, and environmental groups are just a few places to consider. Or you can volunteer to help senior citizens or to read to children.

You can also go on a "volunteer vacation," where volunteers participate in community projects for local people. Projects through the Global Citizen's Volunteer Network can be anything from painting, decorating, or construction to helping out at village clinics and schools in places such as Nepal, Guatemala, or Native American reservations.

Here is a way to start spreading happiness: Look inside your local paper for a weekly listing of needs in the community. Or contact the Volunteers of America (VOA) for information on local, national, and international opportunities. Call their toll-free number at (800) 899-0089 or log on to www.voa.org, www.consciouschoice.com, or www.volunteermatch.org. For volunteer vacations, contact www.globalcitizens.org, or call the Global Citizen's Network toll-free number at (800) 644-9292.

> **—Michele Wheat Dugan** *is a licensed psychologist, a certified hypnotherapist, and a "Dances of Universal Peace" teacher in Kutztown, Pennsylvania.*

REACH OUT AND LEAD A PACK OF WARRIOR WOMEN

Can't find a local support group?
Take the initiative to start your own.
You will benefit in countless ways.

Leading a group can be a real inspiration as it will remind you of your connection with all women. You may discover leadership abilities that will help you and your group to discover who you really are: beautiful, wise, wonderful, powerful women.

Counselor Louise Hay offers some suggestions for those who want to start a support group.

• Create an environment that is safe for deep sharing. Ways to do this include asking everyone to make a commitment to confidentiality and making it clear that the group is a place to let down the masks we often wear. No one is expected to have a perfect life.

• Establish guidelines at the first meeting such as the following: make a commitment to attend all sessions; be respectful of the time and the need to give others a chance to share; do not cross-talk while someone is speaking; focus sharing on the issue, not the whole "story"; try to use responsible language such as using "I" statements like "I feel . . ." rather than "They made me . . ."

• If the group is large, you can have people form small groups of five or six.

• Cultivate a nonjudgmental, accepting attitude. Do not tell anyone what they "should" do. Offer suggestions for ways that they could change their thoughts and perspectives. If people sense judgment, they will immediately go into resistance.

- Each group is different, and each session will be different. Learn to flow with the energy of the current group and session.

- If someone is trying to dominate the group, tell her in private that you appreciate all that she shares with the group, but your concern is that others who are not as assertive may feel inhibited. Finding some task that this woman could assist you with may also be helpful.

- Don't argue with someone who seems to want to stay stuck. Try not to allow yourself to get depressed by someone else's drama. As a group leader, you must learn to hold on to that sense of knowing that healing is available to everyone, whether or not they claim it.

- Develop a sense of humor. Laughter is a marvelous way of gaining a different perspective.

- After each group session, go to the mirror and tell yourself how well you're doing, especially if you are new to leading groups.

- Begin and end each session with a meditation or centering process. It can be as simple as having everyone close their eyes or hold hands and breathe for a moment or two.

—Louise Hay *leads metaphysical study groups and empowerment workshops and is the author of numerous self-growth books, including* Empowering Women: Every Woman's Guide to Successful Living.

LOOK OUT
FOR NUMBER ONE

You may be world's most generous care-giver, but finding ways to indulge yourself is not only well-deserved but also imperative for your well-being.

Mood swings, crying spells, and irritability shouldn't all be chalked up to hormones. Have you stopped to consider your lifestyle? Women of menopausal age have sometimes been called the sandwich generation, caught between the demands of raising their own children and the responsibility of caring for aging or ill parents. Being tugged in so many directions (children, husband, parents, housework, job) often leaves little or no time for the self.

"Self-care replenishes us, restores us. Without that refueling, you can become depleted emotionally and won't be able to take care of anyone, including yourself," says Peggy Elam, Ph.D.

Dr. Elam suggests these delightful nurturing ideas. Schedule in time for opportunities like these, she says.

• If you are always everyone else's sympathetic ear, it's time to be your own, too. Buy a cassette recorder and some audiotapes. Talk into it about the anxiety or confusion you may feel. It literally helps to get worry, anxiety, or frustration out of your head and your body.

• Start a weekly bath ritual. Light some candles or incense and play your favorite relaxing music. Savor a glass of wine or mug of herbal tea while you bask. Afterward, send love and appreciation to each part of your body as you rub it with lotion. This is a little thing, but it can make a marvelous difference in your life.

• Whether it's an attic guest room, the bedroom of a child who has moved out of the house, or a treehouse, claim your own sacred space in the world. Make it beautiful. Hang pictures and paint the walls with colors that inspire you. Bring in plants or flowers. Buy art supplies to play with, and a radio. Into this space, let out the meditation maven, poet, sculptress, storyteller, or spoon player who has always lived latently within you. If you don't have space in your house to devote an entire room to yourself, carve out a corner somewhere, but make sure it's entirely your own.

• Take yourself on a date to a museum, a movie, a garden, the library. Do all the things for yourself that really make you feel loved and content, like buying yourself flowers, picking up roasted chestnuts from a street vendor along the way, or pausing to watch geese pass overhead.

• Play hooky once every few months from work if you have a really stressful job.

• Treat yourself to a country bed-and-breakfast or retreat center for the weekend.

• Learn to say no if you really don't feel like doing something for someone else that day.

—Peggy Elam, Ph.D., *is a clinical psychologist and psychotherapist in Nashville.*

PRAY FOR PEACE

Menopause might be prime time to come into or discover a mature spirituality.

More than 250 published empirical studies in the medical literature show statistical relationships between spiritual practices and positive health outcomes—mental health included. "For many menopausal women, prayer offers a dimension of inner peace that cannot be achieved any other way," says Alice D. Domar, Ph.D.

Sophia, a menopausal patient of Dr. Domar's who was struggling with a deep sense of loss after her four daughters were grown, turned back to her Catholic school roots. Whenever she felt most anxious or alone, Sophia repeated the phrase, "Hail Mary, full of grace."

"Of course, Sophia had to work through many psychological issues in order to handle her losses, strengthen her family relations, and find her own path. But she credits her practice of prayer—above all treatment, even estrogen therapy—for regaining her peace of mind. Over time, not only did Sophia's hot flashes abate (without medication), so did her sense of disconnection and loneliness," says Dr. Domar.

Prayer, of course, comes in many forms. Practice prayer in any way that is comfortable and meaningful for you, given your religious history and proclivities. The bottom line is to do some seeking, says Dr. Domar. Make a commitment to finding your own spiritual perspective and a form of prayer that acknowledges and honors your most personal beliefs.

Science has discovered that it doesn't take a formal or complex prayer to reap health benefits. Studies have shown that simply repeating a sacred or meaningful word or phrase produces a relaxation response. Here are some common focus words or phrases to begin your practice.

Christian

Come, Lord
Lord, have mercy
Our Father, who art in Heaven
Hail Mary, full of grace
The Lord is my shepherd

Jewish

Sh'ma ("Hear, O Israel")
Echod ("One")
Shalom ("Peace")
Hashem ("The Name")
Shekhinah ("The Feminine Face of God")

Eastern

Om (the universal sound)
Shanti ("Peace")

Aramaic

Marantha ("Come, Lord")
Abba ("Father")

Islamic

Allah

—Alice D. Domar, Ph.D., *directs the women's health programs for the division of behavioral medicine at Harvard Medical School. She is an assistant professor of medicine at Harvard Medical School, a staff psychologist at the Beth Israel Deaconess Medical Center, and coauthor of* Self-Nurture.

FIND YOURSELF
IN WOMEN'S LITERATURE

Take yourself to the place where can you
Walk the Long Quiet Highway *in the light*
of your full creativity, learn to demand
from the world **A Room of Your Own,** *and*
release your spirit to **Run With the**
Wolves. *Sound esoteric? It's not.*
It's women's lit.

Share in the vicissitudes and grand transformations of sisters all over the planet through multi-ethnic short-story
anthologies. Invoke your inherent creative force through
Alice Notley's poetry, experience a midlife erotic awakening
along with novelist Edith Wharton, or reinvent a more empowering use of language for yourself through Mary Daly's
feminist writings.

Women's literature brings you into an infinite family of
heroines and may give you the first opportunity in your life
to deeply discuss certain dimensions of womanhood. The
students of writing and literature professor Heather Thomas,
Ph.D., have commented that reading women's literature has
given them a powerful boost to their self-esteem as well as a
newfound sense of groundedness.

Consider signing up for a course in women's literature.
If homework and being graded is too much pressure, ask
to audit the class (participate without being graded). Or
for a less-formal sharing of women's words, consider
starting a women's reading circle. Invite your female
friends, relatives, and colleagues, or post an invitation at

local libraries, grocery stores, coffee shops, and bookstores.

Whether you are making suggestions for your community of readers, expanding on a women's literature class, or are simply browsing your local library, explore this list of works recommended by Dr. Thomas.

Poetry

- *Moving Borders*, edited by Mary Margaret Sloan
- *No More Masks!*, edited by Florence Howe
- *These Are Not Sweet Girls*, edited by Marjorie Agosin
- *Trouble the Water*, edited by Jerry W. Ward Jr.
- *Women in Praise of the Sacred*, edited by Jane Hirschfield

Myth/Psychology

- *Goddesses in Everywoman*, by Jean Shinoda Bolen, M.D.
- *The Woman's Encyclopedia of Myths and Secrets*, edited by Barbara G. Walker
- *Women Who Run With the Wolves*, by Clarissa Pinkola Estes, Ph.D.

Creative Writing

- *Pain and Possibility*, by Gabriele Lusser Rico
- *Writing for Your Life*, by Deena Metzger

Autobiography/Memoir

- *An American Childhood*, by Annie Dillard
- *The Autobiography of Alice B. Toklas*, by Gertrude Stein
- *Coming of Age in Mississippi*, by Anne Moody
- Diaries by Virginia Woolf, Anaïs Nin, May Sarton
- *I Know Why the Caged Bird Sings*, by Maya Angelou
- *Moments of Being*, by Virginia Woolf, second edition, edited by Jeanne Schulkind

- *The Norton Book of Women's Lives*, edited by Phyllis Rose
- *On Women Turning Forty*, with interviews and photographs by Cathleen Rountree
- *The Price of My Soul*, by Bernadette Devlin
- *Prime of Life*, by Simone deBeauvoir
- *Silent Dancing*, by Julia Ortiz Cofer
- *The Woman Warrior*, by Maxine Hong Kingston
- *Writing Women's Lives*, edited by Susan Cahill

Short Fiction

- *Love, Struggle, and Change*, edited by Irene Zahava
- *A Map of Hope*, edited by Marjorie Agosin
- *Wayward Girls and Wicked Women*, edited by Angela Carter
- *Women and Fiction*, edited by Susan Cahill

Drama

- *W;t*, by Margaret Edson, Pulitzer Prize winner (title is spelled *W;t* with a semicolon but pronounced "Wit")

—Heather H. Thomas, Ph.D., *is an English and writing professor at Kutztown University in Pennsylvania and a poet and novelist whose works include* Practicing Amnesia.

Savoring Sex

"Part of the reason for eating right and taking care of my health is not just for my heart, not just for my bones, but also for good sex."

—Patricia Love, Ed.D., *marriage and family therapist and relationship consultant in Austin, Texas, and coauthor of* Hot Monogamy

SMOOTH THE WAY

Sex that leaves you sore is no fun.
Over-the-counter lubricants can
effectively create a climate for pleasure.

You probably never really appreciated estrogen when you had lots of it. Once menopausal symptoms began, though, you missed how well it kept you primed for intimate moments. But there's no need to postpone passion in its absence. Head to the drugstore and pick up some over-the-counter lubricants, recommends Mary Jane Minkin, M.D.

If estrogen decline for you means vaginal dryness and less supple vaginal tissue, even after arousal, Dr. Minkin recommends water-based creams, such as K-Y Jelly and Astroglide. Apply the creams immediately before intercourse.

If you're experiencing discomfort from vaginal dryness throughout the day, you may benefit from a long-lasting cream, such as Replens or K-Y Long Lasting. These are usually applied three times per week to maintain continuous lubrication. Follow package directions.

Estrogen creams and estrogen rings inserted into the vagina can also help restore moisture to dry, tender tissues over time. (They aren't meant to be used during the heat of intercourse, however.) Estrogen creams and rings are available through prescription only, so ask your doctor about risks and benefits if over-the-counter methods are inadequate.

—Mary Jane Minkin, M.D., *is a clinical professor of obstetrics and gynecology at Yale University School of Medicine and coauthor of* What Every Woman Needs to Know about Menopause.

DON'T KEEP YOUR LOVER IN THE DARK

When menopausal symptoms leave you less than lustful, it's essential to discuss solutions with your partner.

Does intercourse suddenly make you wince? Whether your sex life is being compromised by painful intercourse, low energy, fragile emotions, or any other of the many complications of menopause hormonal changes, don't bottle up your desires. Denying your passionate nature saps one of the most sublime pleasures from life—not to mention your mate's.

Avoiding sex could very well be misinterpreted as rejection by your lover, warns Peggy Elam, Ph.D. You have enough stress to manage during menopause without straining your most intimate, supporting relationship. By bringing your issues to the table as early on as possible, you are protecting your partner from confusion and pain—and protecting yourself from unnecessary isolation.

Be especially careful of what you say immediately after an unpleasant encounter. A conversation tinged with feelings of shame, frustration, or even anger won't produce a positive outcome, advises Dr. Elam. Instead, choose a private, somewhat neutral spot for your conversation. It's usually best to talk about sex outside the bedroom, like during a relaxing car ride.

When you do broach the subject, let your partner know right up front that you are approaching or going through menopause. Make it clear that physical changes, not your affection, are affecting your lovemaking.

Once you have opened up the lines of communication, you can experiment with solutions. Perhaps, for example, he needs to understand that at midlife a woman requires a longer period of foreplay, and you can learn seductive massage techniques together. Many remedies for your specific concerns are addressed in this chapter, but you may be delightfully surprised to discover what the two of you can come up with on your own. Once he knows that vaginal dryness is a nuisance, together you can make using lubrication part of the fun. Maybe he'll finally take you on that romance-revving lingerie shopping date that he's been procrastinating about for 30 years of marriage.

The fact is, for many women, menopause becomes a liberating time to experiment with different sexual behaviors, such as oral sex. Communicate—and you're on the road to joining the ranks of women who report their postmenopausal years as their best sex years.

—Peggy Elam, Ph.D., *is a clinical psychologist and psychotherapist in Nashville.*

EXPERIENCE AN X-RATED EVENING

While you're going through the change, changing an off-limits attitude toward risqué films can help fan your fires.

If you're spending too many nights renting *Star Trek* videos rather than shooting off your own rockets, you and your lover might consider a more arousing form of entertainment. Films with steamy love scenes, particularly those depicting the kind of characters you can relate to, can turn up the heat for menopausal women who experience low libidos, according to Barbara D. Bartlik, M.D.

Since your estrogen and testosterone levels wane as you age, you may encounter diminished sensitivity in your breasts and genital area, often increasing the amount of time it takes to feel sexually aroused. The bottom line is that many women require more intense forms of stimulation, and that's where erotic films can help. Erotic images actually flood the body with some of the same hormones that sex does. Not only can torrid love scenes excite sexual feelings, they can introduce you to new, possibly more enjoyable methods for achieving fulfillment, says Dr. Bartlik.

Unlike pornography, the type of film you might want to seek out, as a mature woman, is from the "erotica" category of adult entertainment. Good erotica films feature respectable characters in sensitive, sexually charged relationships. If you're scanning the video shelves looking for a little sophistication, select films produced by women and those depicting more mature couples on the cover, says Dr.

Bartlik. Keep in mind also that films featuring characters with less "model-like" bodies will help you connect to the action better than those targeted to a younger audience.

Videos that have a menopausal woman's needs in mind can be discreetly purchased online or through mail order. The Femme Productions company, for example, uniquely offers films written and produced by women and claims to promote a softer, more sensual approach to erotic film by tapping into a woman's version of sexual fantasy. To purchase a video, contact Candida Royalle's Femme online at www.royalle.com, or call (800) 456-LOVE for a catalog.

Dr. Bartlik also recommends educational films produced by the Sinclair Intimacy Institute. These explicit guides, such as the best-selling *Better Sex Series*, are hosted by medical professionals and sex therapists. Some feature special sexual concerns of over-40 and over-50 viewers, while others discuss and actually demonstrate new intimacy situations that you may wish to explore. That series is available online at www.intimacyinstitute.com, or call (800) 955-0888, ext. 8NET2, for a catalog.

—Barbara D. Bartlik, M.D., *is a clinical assistant professor in the department of psychiatry at Weill Medical College of Cornell University and assistant attending psychiatrist at the New York Presbyterian Hospital, both in New York City.*

E-LIMINATE DRYNESS NATURALLY

Vexed by painful intercourse as a result of vaginal dryness? Daily doses of vitamin E can foster that missing moisture.

Vitamin E is a longtime remedy recommended by natural health practitioners to treat vaginal atrophy (thinning and drying of the vaginal lining). Vitamin E seems to do the work that your body's own estrogen did when you were younger, to restore the lubrication of the vaginal lining, says Tori Hudson, N.D.

Dr. Hudson recommends taking 400 IU of vitamin E daily to fortify your tender tissue. But don't stop there, she says. You can insert a gelatin capsule of vitamin E (soft or hard style, it doesn't matter) directly into your vagina. The oil will gradually be absorbed into the vaginal wall. Do that once or twice a day, depending on the severity of dryness, for 1 month. Over time, your vagina will become more supple and moist, Dr. Hudson says. After a month, you can reduce your application to two or three times per week.

Combining the topical treatment with the 400 IU oral supplement is safe and may be continued indefinitely, she says. If you are taking aspirin or a blood-thinning medication, however, check with your doctor before supplementing, because vitamin E will compound the effects of the anticoagulants.

—Tori Hudson, N.D., *is a professor at the National College of Naturopathic Medicine and the medical director of A Woman's Time clinic, both in Portland, Oregon. She is the author of* The Women's Encyclopedia of Natural Medicine.

LUBRICATE WITH LICORICE

*A daily dose of licorice can keep you
more comfortable during the day and
more amorous at night.*

Although licorice is better known for treating coughs and ulcers, natural health care professionals have also found that it does wonders for toning the mucous membranes of the reproductive system as well. "When tender vaginal tissue needs to be moister—a common complaint of women during and after menopause—licorice is a choice remedy," according to Helen Healy, N.D. She's even had patients in their eighties benefit.

Unlike topically applied lubricants, which are quickly absorbed back into the vaginal tissue, licorice is believed to imitate the role of estrogen in the body, activating the production of mucus and helping to "plump up" the thinning vaginal wall, says Dr. Healy. For that reason, it's a good remedy for women who forgo hormone-replacement therapy (HRT). (Those who take HRT shouldn't need licorice.)

She suggests using only deglycyrrhizinated licorice, labeled DGL. Whole licorice can stimulate the adrenal glands, which aggravates hypertension and could create serious risks, especially in aging women. Tablets marked DGL provide the benefits without those risks.

Begin by taking two 380-milligram tablets of the dried herb three times daily to keep the vaginal area moist throughout the day, she says. Once the vaginal tissue is fortified, you might find fewer tablets are necessary. Use it as long as needed.

—Helen Healy, N.D., *a naturopathic physician, is the director of the Wellspring Naturopathic Clinic in St. Paul, Minnesota.*

SOOTHE YOUR SINUSES, SAVE YOUR SEX LIFE

The antihistamines you take to relieve your nose and eyes during the allergy season may stifle sexual comfort.

Antihistamines can be a big help during allergy season. They dry out the mucous membranes in your sinuses so you can get through the day without being bleary-eyed and sniffly. Trouble is, these drugs also rob moisture from the lining of your vagina.

That's especially bad during and after menopause, when ebbing estrogen levels leave the lower regions less lubricated. Without adequate lubrication, you'll experience an unpleasant friction during intercourse. So, it's best not to take antihistamines if vaginal dryness is a problem, says Tori Hudson, N.D.

As an alternative to antihistamine drugs, Dr. Hudson suggests substituting the nutritional supplement quercetin, a bioflavonoid derived from citrus fruits and buckwheat. Rather than drying out your body, quercetin goes to work on the cells that release histamines, stabilizing them and preventing such reactions as watery eyes and runny noses. Quercetin is available in tablet form from health food stores and drugstores.

Dr. Hudson recommends taking 200 to 400 milligrams of quercetin three times per day, between meals, through allergy season. It is considered safe, with no side effects.

—Tori Hudson, N.D., *is a professor at the National College of Naturopathic Medicine and the medical director of A Woman's Time clinic, both in Portland, Oregon. She is the author of* The Women's Encyclopedia of Natural Medicine.

KEEP UP WITH CONTRACEPTION

When it comes to birth control, better safe than sorry is a rule not to break when you're approaching menopause.

Sex without risk of pregnancy could make those annoying menopausal symptoms seem worthwhile. But don't toss your contraceptives away after your first hot flash. "Pregnancy is possible during the perimenopausal years," warns Brian Walsh, M.D. "Admittedly, the risk is low, but it's not zero."

An unplanned pregnancy on the brink of menopause could prove both physically and emotionally burdensome, so it's essential to use birth control every time you have intercourse. Since irregular menstrual cycles make it difficult to judge "safe" times, the rhythm method is unreliable.

Barrier methods, which include diaphragms and condoms, are wise choices, says Dr. Walsh. Spermicidal formulas, however, can irritate sensitive vaginal tissue and should be avoided if vaginal dryness, typical of menopause, is a problem. Women who can safely take estrogen may benefit from low-dose birth control pills, which also offer symptomatic relief from hot flashes and menstrual irregularities.

When do contraceptives become extraneous? After your periods have stopped completely for 1 year, says Dr. Walsh. Since on-again-off-again cycles can make the determination difficult, it's best to consult with your doctor before stopping.

—Brian Walsh, M.D., *is an assistant professor of obstetrics and gynecology and reproductive biology at Harvard Medical School and the director of the Menopause Clinic at Brigham and Women's Hospital, both in Boston.*

GET A NEW ANGLE
ON PLEASURE

If recurrent urinary tract infections are taking a toll on your sex life, you may need to revise your lovemaking style.

For some women, it's a fact of life. Once menopause hits, they get slammed with more urinary tract infections (UTIs). Trying a new maneuver in bed could actually reduce the risk of infections, says Domeena C. Renshaw, M.D.

As estrogen levels dip during menopause, the walls of the vagina become thinner, leaving less protection between it and the tube leading from the bladder, called the urethra. During intercourse, the penis can bump the urethra against the bony bridge of the pelvis, creating an uncomfortable sensation and pushing bacteria into the urethral opening. Once bacteria finds its way in, an infection can take hold, says Dr. Renshaw. Symptoms include a frequent urge to urinate, painful burning during urination, and urine that is cloudy or tinged with blood.

To prevent UTIs, Dr. Renshaw recommends using the L-shaped position when you have intercourse. This is done with the man and woman lying on their sides, facing one another. The woman lifts her upper leg and the man slides his upper leg beneath it. The penis enters the vagina at a sideways angle so that it doesn't pound against the opening of the urethra, explains Dr. Renshaw.

—Domeena C. Renshaw, M.D., *is a professor and assistant chairperson in the department of psychiatry and the director of the Sexual Dysfunction Clinic at the Loyola University Medical Center in Chicago.*

BUY YOURSELF
A MAGIC WAND

*If you've had a long lapse from sexual
relations, a dilator may be invaluable.*

It's not unusual for postmenopausal woman to experience
a narrowing of the vagina that prevents penetration, particularly if she has spent years without a partner. Fortunately, a vaginal dilator can retrain her anatomy for a sexual
relationship.

A dilator is a smooth glass wand that is inserted manu-
ally into the vagina on a daily basis for anywhere from 1 to
6 months, according to Brian Walsh, M.D. In cases of severe
narrowing, a patient may need to gradually increase the size
of the dilator over a period of months. Once the muscles are
widened, the condition will not return as long as regular intercourse is resumed.

A long hiatus from sex can also heighten the effects of
vaginal atrophy common among menopausal women. Atrophy is characterized by drying and thinning of tissues in
and around the vagina, making it prone to infection and
easily irritated. To offset those symptoms, dilators are normally used in conjunction with topical estrogen creams,
which enable the vagina to produce natural secretions and
improve suppleness. Both dilators and estrogen creams are
available by prescription only.

—Brian Walsh, M.D., *is an assistant professor of obstet-
rics and gynecology and reproductive biology at Harvard
Medical School and the director of the Menopause Clinic at
Brigham and Women's Hospital, both in Boston.*

PUT A NEW SLANT ON GREAT SEX

Keep the muscles in your pubic region toned with Kegel exercises, and maximize results by doing them on an incline.

As women age, their uterine muscles tend to weaken and sag downward, undermining full sensations of intercourse or even causing the embarrassment of leaking urine in the heat of the moment. But you can battle gravity by keeping the supporting muscles toned with daily Kegel exercises, says Helen Healy, N.D. For the best results, do them while lying on a slantboard, a padded exercise board set on an adjustable incline.

Kegel exercises consist of contracting and relaxing the pubococcygeal muscles, which are used to stop and start the flow of urine. When those muscles are in good working order, the tissues surrounding them remain healthier and better oxygenated, says Dr. Healy. By strengthening them, menopausal women can maintain better control and even better vaginal lubrication. Better yet, women report improved sex lives and more intense orgasms after doing Kegels routinely.

Dr. Healy suggests lying on a slantboard set at a 25- to 30-degree angle (with one end raised about 2 feet) with your head at the low end. While in that position, squeeze the pubococcygeal muscles hard and hold them for about 5 seconds, then release and relax for 3 seconds. Always do this on an empty stomach to prevent a potential hiatal hernia. For optimum benefits, work up to 100 squeezes per day. Not all of these need to be done on a slantboard. The beauty of

Kegels is that you can pretty much do them anywhere, and no one will know it, she says.

Slantboards can usually be purchased wherever exercise equipment is sold. If you're on a tight budget, you can create your own slantboard by carefully propping up and securing one end of a padded ironing board on a sofa seat, bench, or stool.

> **—Helen Healy, N.D.,** *a naturopathic physician, is the director of the Wellspring Naturopathic Clinic in St. Paul, Minnesota.*

EAT YOGURT, STARVE YEAST

Don't trade one infection for another. When you are being treated for a bacterial infection with antibiotics, adding yogurt to your menu could avoid the nasty yeast backlash.

After menopause, your vagina loses some of its protective lining. That means it becomes more easily abraded and more prone to bacterial and yeast infections, which cause itching, irritation, and, often, pain during intercourse. Sex turns into a turnoff.

Oral antibiotics take care of the bacterial infections, but they can actually lead to more vaginal yeast infections—at a time when you're already more vulnerable, according to Loren G. Lipson, M.D. Why the complications? Oral antibiotics are formulated to fight bacteria throughout the body, and unfortunately in the process, they also annihilate the beneficial ones in the reproductive tract. As a result, the normally small, harmless population of yeast that resides in the reproductive canals can increase wildly.

Most yogurt contains beneficial bacteria in the form of acidophilus and bifidus (often labeled as "active cultures"). When populations of these active cultures are high enough, they suppress yeast.

To fight off yeast naturally, treat yourself to at least one 8-ounce serving of yogurt a day. Check the label; the yogurt must contain live acidophilus and bifidus cultures. Yogurt with the least sugar is best since sugar seems to encourage yeast. If yogurt doesn't agree with you, try taking acidophilus and bifidus supplements, available as drops or tablets from health food stores. Follow package directions for dosage amounts. Take supplements at least 2 hours after the antibiotic. Otherwise, you'll risk killing off the bacteria in the supplement. If you have any serious gastrointestinal problems that require medical attention, check with your doctor before taking the supplement.

Active cultures can be taken in conjunction with over-the-counter anti-yeast suppositories and creams, says Dr. Lipson. If a yeast infection persists for more than 1 week, it's important to see your doctor for proper treatment and diagnosis.

—Loren G. Lipson, M.D., *is an associate professor of medicine and chief of the division of geriatric medicine at the University of Southern California in Los Angeles.*

MAKE LOVE MORE

*Frequent sex in midlife and beyond is
good for you and can even help manage
some symptoms of menopause.*

According to the results of a University of Chicago study,
women who engage in sex once a week have higher estrogen levels. In fact, women with sporadic, rather than
weekly sexual activity, had a 50 percent chance of developing severely low estrogen levels. The benefit of consistent
indulging may very well translate to fewer hot flashes, less
vaginal dryness, better withstanding osteoporosis, and aging
more slowly, says Patricia Love, Ed.D.

The specific reasons that sex is good for keeping aging
women youthful are a bit complex, says Dr. Love. It all begins with oxytocin, the chemical that triggers orgasm (also
released during breastfeeding) and causes you to bond with
your partner, she explains. Bonding encourages more
touching, and that, in turn, releases endorphins, the body's
natural "opiates." When this happens often, Dr. Love says
that it colors your life with a sense of tranquillity and happiness that ultimately offsets aging, both emotionally and
physically.

Dr. Love suggests maintaining weekly sexual relations
even if you don't always feel like it. "You might just think of
sex as meeting your partner's needs. What you don't realize
is that it's also good for you because it sends a signal to your
body that says, 'I'm still young, alive, and vibrant,'" she says.

Not motivated this week? If you're even neutral and he's
willing, experts recommend letting him start the action. Remember all those times that once the buttons came undone,
you ended up even surprising yourself with how feral you

felt? If you still feel untouchable but aren't opposed to intimacy, doing some "favors" for him also boosts your hormone levels.

Another dividend: Regular sexual activity stimulates the
vaginal lining to produce natural lubricants, keeping vaginal
dryness at bay. And if your own lubrication is inadequate,
sex encourages you to apply creams and moisturizers, which
further maintains vaginal health. To reap that benefit, you
don't need a partner. Masturbating twice a week can produce
the same results.

> **—Patricia Love, Ed.D.,** *is a marriage and family therapist
> and relationship consultant in Austin, Texas, and coauthor of*
> Hot Monogamy.

PAMPER YOURSELF CAREFULLY

*Using feminine personal-care products
may be a favorite way to celebrate your
womanhood. But in the long run, you
may just end up irritated.*

Bath oils, bubbles, deodorant soaps, douches, decorative
toilet tissue, and even some laundry detergents can
trigger discomfort in your delicate vaginal tissues—a particular concern for menopausal women, according to Mary
Jane Minkin, M.D.

Before the onset of menopause, the hormone estrogen
keeps your vagina lubricated, which protects it from poten-
tially irritating substances. But as estrogen levels start to

drop, the mucous membranes of your vagina become thinner and less moist. Soaps, which wash away your body's protective oils, only enhance that drying effect, increasing the likelihood of painful intercourse. What's more, once damaged by irritants, thin vaginal tissues are more prone to yeast and bacterial infections, another source of sexual discomfort.

Deodorant soaps, which usually contain perfumes and dyes, can be especially hard on sensitive tissue. Two milder brands that Dr. Minkin recommends are Dove (white only) and Neutrogena. When it comes to baths, soaking in a tub of soapy bubbles or scented oils is an invitation for irritation. Showers are best, but oatmeal baths, or even daily baths without added soaps, are also okay.

As for laundry detergents, it's best to stick to the brand your body's used to. But if you notice irritation, switch to something without scents or bleaching agents. Flush your affection for decorative or colored toilet tissue as well, she says. Always use an undyed or white variety, since dyes are potential irritants. And definitely don't douche, Dr. Minkin says. Douching further strips your vagina of natural lubricants.

—Mary Jane Minkin, M.D., *is a clinical professor of obstetrics and gynecology at Yale University School of Medicine and coauthor of* What Every Woman Needs to Know about Menopause.

INDULGE IN HERBAL APHRODISIACS

Certain herbs have been reputed throughout history to pep up passion. Combining two of the best-known menopause helpers might double your pleasure.

The Mexican herb damiana has a widely established folk reputation for enlivening the feminine libido. Experts don't agree on whether or not it's medically warranted as an aphrodisiac, but the herb is generally accepted for its ability to stabilize your emotions. Because of the herb's mild mood-enhancement abilities, herbal expert David Winston recommends damiana when he hears women complain of low libido. The theory is that since the herb can curb your anxiety levels and lift you out of the doldrums, your lovin' feelings have more chance to flourish.

Winston prescribes damiana in conjunction with the herb chasteberry (also known as vitex), which helps normalize the female hormonal system. Since it helps regulate estrogen levels and may increase progesterone production, chasteberry may not only increase a woman's appetite for sex but also control hot flashes and vaginal dryness.

Both herbs are available in health food stores and are considered safe for long-term use, says Winston. Damiana can be taken in tea form. Pour 8 ounces of boiling water over 1 teaspoon of the dried herb. Cover and steep it for 40 minutes. Strain and drink 4 ounces three times a day. If you prefer, take two capsules of the dried herb three times a day.

Take one 40-milligram capsule of chasteberry twice a day or 40 to 60 drops of the tincture twice a day. Chasteberry may counteract the effects of birth control pills. Do not use during pregnancy.

—**David Winston** *is a founding member of the American Herbalists Guild and is president of Herbalist and Alchemist Inc., an herbalist training school and herbal production company in Washington, New Jersey.*

STAY ON TOP OF OSTEOPOROSIS

Sex can't be gratifying if it means putting painful pressure on frail bones threatened or damaged by osteoporosis. Taking the lead in sex will ensure your safety and comfort.

Estrogen plays many roles in keeping your body functioning, and maintaining bone density is one of them. As a result of estrogen's waning, your risk of developing osteoporosis increases once you hit menopause.

In the advanced stages of osteoporosis, the bones in your spine can become so weak that they break, literally, with a sneeze. These fractures are painful and take a long time to heal. What's more, bones elsewhere in your body are also more fragile and susceptible to breaks, especially the hips and wrists.

Having sex while lying on your back with the full weight

of your partner on top can be both dangerous and painful if you have brittle bones. But just because the missionary position is uncomfortable does not mean that you have to take a vow of celibacy. Instead, climbing on top could take you back into the pleasure zone.

"If you want to avoid pain, the woman-on-top position may help because you have more control," explains Domeena C. Renshaw, M.D.

The most basic method is to lie over your partner; this is called a reverse missionary position when the woman is on top. Or you can sit up and straddle his pelvis, unless of course, you have knee pain. In that case, continue to experiment with positions where you are on top. Dr. Renshaw reminds couples to maintain a sense of humor and adventure about testing new positions and to communicate about what feels pleasurable for both.

—Domeena C. Renshaw, M.D., *is a professor and assistant chairperson in the department of psychiatry and the director of the Sexual Dysfunction Clinic at the Loyola University Medical Center in Chicago.*

Alternative Options

Alternative practitioners' compassionate attention to your overall well-being is the kind of care that can benefit your long-term health and happiness as you pass through the many stages of maturity. The preventive focus of alternative medicine can help you to avoid menopausal health problems altogether. But if needs do arise, expect a unique array of nondrug methods for gentle menopausal symptom relief.

Unlike taking a pill, your prescription from an alternative health practitioner is likely to be a highly personalized program, based on your individual symptoms, history, and desires. Expect practitioners to include you in decisions about what treatments fit, since they traditionally value the role that your mind and spirit play in the healing process.

Be alert when reading this guide as to which methods, in particular, appeal to you. Are you drawn to biofeedback to ease hormonal headaches, herbs to reduce hot flashes, or massage to decrease insomnia? Are you intrigued by the idea of a yoga teacher teaching you ancient poses that lessen depression and anxiety?

If you are still unsure where to start, your best bet is to visit a naturopathic physician or holistic gynecologist. These practitioners are skilled in the widest variety of natural therapy options.

Biofeedback Practitioners

Biofeedback relies on the power of your mind as well as tools of the high-tech age to help you smoothly make the transition through menopause. Practitioners say that it can mute a host of problems associated with menopause, including insomnia, attention problems, mood changes, hot flashes, and headaches.

Typically, during a biofeedback session, electrodes are attached to your skin. These sensors monitor body functions such as temperature, muscle tension, brain wave activity, and heart rate. Even the slightest change in any one of these can be detected by a biofeedback machine and turned into a signal that you can see or hear. With this feedback and a bit of coaching from your biofeedback practitioner, you can learn to calm your brain and body functions.

To get the best results from biofeedback, you'll need to practice with a professional for 10 to 40 sessions. One sign of competent training is a practitioner's certification by the Biofeedback Certification Institute of America.

To find a biofeedback practitioner in your area, send a self-addressed, stamped envelope (SASE) to: The Biofeedback Certification Institute of America, 10200 West 44th Avenue, Suite 310, Wheat Ridge, CO 80033, or visit their Web site at www.bcia.org.

Holistic Gynecologists and Holistic Nurse Practitioners

In order to create a well-rounded treatment program for you, holistic gynecologists and nurse practitioners will meld the tools of conventional women's health care with knowledge of nutrition, bodywork, and other natural healing methods.

A holistic gynecologist is a medical doctor (M.D.) who pursues additional training in natural therapies over and above her medical school degree and specialty training in gynecology. If a holistic gynecologist uses this title, she wants to communicate that she respects traditional approaches to women's health care as well as alternative, nondrug methods.

A nurse practitioner (N.P.) has advanced training that allows her to diagnose and treat patients, a task that is usually beyond the scope of a registered nurse (R.N.). Some nurse practitioners have private practices, and others work for doctors. Nurse practitioners are reputed to spend more time with patients than conventional doctors do, which in itself is holistic. But if she adds the word *holistic* to her title, she wishes to also communicate her additional training and commitment to the same alternative health methods as holistic gynecologists.

These specialists often emphasize dietary advice to prevent menopause-associated disease and symptoms. A typical holistic diet for menopausal patients includes high amounts of fiber, omega-3 fatty acids, soy foods, flaxseed; moderate to high amounts of protein; and little saturated fat. Your practitioner may also emphasize yoga, aerobic exercise, and strength training as ways of preventing future disease. She may also refer you to chiropractors, massage therapists, psychotherapists, meditation teachers, or support groups who can help with your individual mind-body concerns—and may provide some of these services herself.

To receive a list of holistic gynecologists in your area, request a directory from the American Holistic Medical Association, 6728 Old McLean Village Drive, McLean, VA 22101, or log on to www.holisticmedicine.org. You can contact the American Holistic Nurses' Association by writing to AHNA, P.O. Box 2130, Flagstaff, AZ 86003-2130, or log on to www.ahna.org.

Massage Therapists

Stress can increase your vulnerability to countless health problems, including those related to menopause. If tension is triggering symptoms, you are in good hands with a massage therapist. Some practitioners can further foster your treatment by combining bodywork with their training in aromatherapy.

More than 100 types of massage and bodywork are available in the United States. Swedish massage, the predominant form, utilizes a combination of nine massage strokes ranging from light touch to deep muscle work. Often, it is done in a softly lit room as soothing music plays in the background. Scented oils may be applied to the skin as well.

"Massage therapy can relieve anxiety, release pent-up emotions, and subdue insomnia, depression, and other menopausal symptoms. But massage therapy also is invigorating," says Beth Miller, a massage therapist and aromatherapy practitioner in North Miami Beach, Florida. As a result, you may be more prone to exercise, which is essential to stave off menopause-related conditions such as osteoporosis and heart disease.

A qualified massage therapist should have completed training at an accredited school. To find a qualified massage therapist, including those who do aromatherapy, contact the American Massage Therapy Association, 820 Davis Street, Suite 100, Evanston, IL 60201, or visit their Web site at www.amtamassage.org.

Naturopathic Physicians

Naturopathic physicians have the advanced training that you may want for many complex menopausal issues, especially balancing your hormones, bucking your genetic predisposition to age-related disease, or easing your emotions. Since naturopaths have been trained in everything from advanced nutrition and herbs to natural hormones and bodywork, they can create the complete program of therapies that works best for you.

"We have both breadth and depth of knowledge," says Tori Hudson, N.D., professor at the National College of Naturopathic Medicine and medical director of A Woman's Time clinic, both in Portland, Oregon, and author of *The Women's Encyclopedia of Natural Medicine*. A qualified naturopath has 4 years of instruction in anatomy, disease, natural medicines, and alternative therapies from an accredited school, including more than 2 years of clinical training.

If you are seeking natural alternatives to synthetic hormone-replacement therapy, a naturopathic physician can determine your levels of estrogens, progesterone, testosterone, and DHEA and recommend a method with the fewest side effects and health risks for you.

"I prefer plant-based hormones because they are biochemically identical to the hormones already in the human body. They have fewer side effects than more conventional synthetic hormones or those that are not biochemically identical to human hormones, such as those derived from animal urine," Dr. Hudson says.

Naturopaths offer specialized formulations of herbs and supplements, which are often unavailable at health food stores. These combinations can help reduce health risks such as high cholesterol, diabetes, osteoporosis, and even cancers.

A qualified naturopath should be a member of the American Association of Naturopathic Physicians (AANP) or the American Naturopathic Association (ANA). Both have specific training requirements.

You can request a directory of naturopathic physicians from the American Association of Naturopathic Physicians (AANP), 8201 Greensboro Drive, Suite 300, McLean, VA 22102, or visit the American Naturopathic Association (ANA) Web site at www.naturopathic.org for more information.

Oriental Medicine Specialists

Oriental medicine is one of the oldest forms of healing and prevention practiced today. Acupuncture has been used in China since at least 400 B.C. and Chinese herbalism since 200 B.C. Having effectively served millions of people throughout the Far East for thousands of years, it's no wonder the demand and number of practitioners is catching on in the Western world, too.

The goal of Traditional Chinese Medicine is to foster health by balancing energy, which is understood in terms of meridians—pathways within the body thought to regulate the body's vital life force or *chi* (pronounced "chee"). There are 12 intersecting energetic meridians, controlled by different organ systems.

Practitioners consider menopausal health problems to be imbalances of the spleen, liver, and kidney energies, which control the reproductive cycle. You may choose from more than a dozen types of Oriental bodywork used to restore this balance, such as the pushing and stretching movements of Thai massage. Acupuncturists insert hair-thin acupuncture needles at points on the meridians thought to increase spleen, liver, or kidney energy, while acupressurists or shiatsu therapists will rub these points with their hands.

"Not only does stimulating meridian points help specific symptoms, such as hot flashes, it generally gives a woman more stamina and helps her sleep better," says Claudette Baker, L.Ac., licensed acupuncturist and Chinese herbalist in Evanston, Illinois.

Bodywork is only one dimension of the mosaic of Oriental medicine practiced by a full doctor of Oriental medicine (O.M.D. or T.C.M.). These doctors create individualized programs with dietary modifications, exercise, and meditation. Oriental doctors may also prescribe Chinese herbs that can be taken as powders, granules, or teas, which they often mix themselves to suit a patient's individual needs.

To find a qualified Oriental medicine specialist in your area, contact the American Association of Oriental Medicine, 433 Front Street, Catasauqua, PA 18032. For bodywork in particular, contact the American Oriental Bodywork Therapies of Asia at 1010 Haddonfield-Berlin Road, Suite 408, Voorhees, NJ 08043, or log on to www.aobta.org.

Yoga Instructors

A regular yoga practice helps women maintain their well-being by deepening their sense of self, explains Svaroopa yoga instructor Linda Rado of West Reading, Pennsylvania. She finds that students who enter menopause after years of consistent yoga practice are less affected by physical and emotional turbulence.

But it's never to late to be supported by yoga's many benefits to your mind, body, and spirit. "Any level of yoga practice can help to balance out hormones and alleviate symptoms," says Trisha Lamb Feuerstein, director of research at the Yoga Research and Education Center in Lower Lake, California.

A qualified yoga instructor can show you specific breathing techniques to control hot flashes, blood pressure, and anxiety. As you progress, she will also teach the headstand and handstand. These inverted poses are beneficial during menopause because they are thought to nourish your thyroid, lower blood pressure, and control sweating by widening blood vessels.

Another dimension of yoga practice are spine twists. These delightful poses not only tone your back but also boost your production of hormones, which can bolster a flagging sex drive and create positive feelings.

As you might expect, the relaxation effects of yoga can

also make your physical and emotional transitions easier. Your teacher may lead you in forward bending poses that calm your nervous system. She can also guide you in achieving a peaceful state of mind through meditation and other techniques such as chanting and breathwork.

Yoga also helps guard against osteoporosis, says Feuerstein. It's one of the few weight-bearing exercises to work on the upper body, producing stronger, denser bones, despite your declining estrogen levels.

Always question a potential yoga teacher about her education. If you have physical injuries or health risks like high blood pressure or osteoporosis, it is especially important to work with a teacher who has advanced training that covers such issues. Training centers and yoga styles known for their knowledge of and attention to special health issues include Integrative Yoga Therapy Centers, Phoenix Rising Yoga Therapy, Kripalu yoga, Svaroopa yoga, Viniyoga, and Iyengar yoga.

To locate a yoga teacher or identify the form that's best for you, contact the Yoga Research and Education Center, P.O. Box 1386, Lower Lake, CA 95457, or log on to www.yrec.org.

For more information on these and other alternative healing modalities, contact the National Center for Complementary and Alternative Medicine at the National Institutes of Health (NIH). Write for their "General Information Package" at NCCAM Clearinghouse, P.O. Box 8218, Silver Spring, MD 20907, or log on to http://nccam.nih.gov.

Index